COVID
BABIES

COVID
BABIES

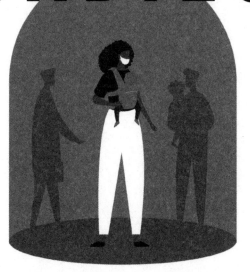

AMY BROWN

Covid Babies: How pandemic health measures undermined pregnancy, birth and early parenting

First published in the UK by Pinter & Martin Ltd 2021

ISBN 978-1-78066-760-7

Also available as an ebook

Edited by Susan Last
Index by Helen Bilton

British Library Cataloguing-in-Publication Data
A catalogue record for this book is available from the British Library

Printed in Poland by Hussar

This book has been printed on paper that is sourced and harvested from sustainable forests and is FSC accredited

Pinter & Martin Ltd
6 Effra Parade
London SW2 1PS

pinterandmartin.com

CONTENTS

INTRODUCTION

It is undeniable that we were all affected by the global Covid-19 pandemic and measures to contain it. Some of us experienced physical health threats to ourselves and our families, with many suffering the loss of much-loved family members. Others had their livelihoods, businesses, and jobs decimated by lockdown measures and changes in priorities. Many struggled with social isolation and loneliness at a time when they needed contact and connection the most. Most likely many of us experienced a combination of these, and we know that the pandemic will have long-lasting repercussions beyond the physical impact of the virus.

On the evening of 23 March 2020, a UK lockdown was imposed with the majority of public places closing, travel restricted and meeting up with others from outside your own household largely prohibited. Over the following 18 months (and most likely beyond) the UK and other countries around the world have seen various implementation and easing of different restrictions around movement, social contact and monitoring of health symptoms.[1]

It soon became clear that the virus was airborne and could spread pretty rapidly between people through infected particles coughed, sneezed or otherwise breathed out. Although the individual risk to people who were younger and without any underlying health conditions was relatively low, those who were older and had health conditions that made it more difficult for them to fight the virus were at greater risk. Whole books could be written on 'how much risk' (and we'll come back to this in the next chapter specifically in relation to pregnant women), but we knew the virus could cause serious harm. Even when an individual's risk is fairly low, if you multiply that by a population of over 66 million, significant numbers of people can become seriously unwell. Obviously that is undesirable from a compassionate perspective, but there was also a risk that if too many people rapidly became unwell at the same time, our healthcare systems would be overwhelmed.

Measures were therefore put in place that essentially aimed to reduce how much contact people had with each other and therefore how likely the virus was to spread. Simplistically, if you limit interactions between people, you limit opportunities for the virus to hop from one person to another, and another, and so on. Of course, some 'contacts' would always be necessary in terms of emergency healthcare, shopping and apparently things like trips out to historical attractions to check your eyesight. But it appeared a hard line was drawn between what the government and advisors deemed 'necessary contacts' and what many people deemed 'necessary' for their wellbeing and mental health. And this is where things really got challenging.

I am not going to comment on the 'necessity' or 'logic' of the restrictions put in place, in part because I am not an epidemiologist, virologist or public health practitioner and therefore don't consider myself qualified to do so. But also (hopefully) we are now at a stage where we are moving forward. There's not a lot we can do to change what has already happened – but we can examine its impact and look at how we can focus our efforts on helping those most affected.

It is clear that the pandemic has had both direct and indirect effects on health – and the ultimate question will be which of these has had the most impact in the longer term. Some people's health was of course directly affected by contracting the virus. However, there were many adverse indirect health and social effects caused by the measures introduced to contain the virus. For example, healthcare (particularly routine and non-emergency appointments) was significantly affected. An article published in the *BMJ* in February 2021 highlighted that the number of patients waiting for planned surgery or surgical care had hit record highs at the end of 2020, with over 6.76 million waiting in the UK. The reasons for this include operating theatres and clinics being used for Covid-19 patients, redeployment of medical and nursing staff, and high levels of infection or isolation requirements among NHS professionals. Additionally, six million fewer patients were referred into consultant-led elective care in 2020 compared to 2019.[2]

These figures do not include the impact of the 'second wave' and what has happened since then. Significantly more patients were admitted to hospital with Covid-19 as the virus progressed. At one point on 18 January 2021 there were over 34,000 Covid-19 patients in English hospitals alone. Obviously these patients needed to be somewhere, and to be treated with finite resources and cared for by a relatively static workforce – it's difficult to magic medical and nursing staff out of thin air, especially when other countries are also in crisis, and the atmosphere is somewhat hostile due to the recent divorce from your European neighbours.[3]

It is also now clear what a significant mental health impact the pandemic has had on many of us. In terms of general wellbeing within the population, data from the Office for National Statistics showed a rapid fall within the first two months of lockdown, falling to the lowest levels ever recorded.[4] A rapid rise in clinical mental health issues has also been seen, with the pandemic both exacerbating existing issues and creating new ones.[5] At the time of writing the NHS is facing record levels of demand for mental health support[6] – which unfortunately it is struggling to meet due to continued underfunding and reductions in space and staff.[7]

While certain demographic groups were statistically at greater health risk from the virus, others appeared to be at greater social and emotional risk from the measures put in place to contain it. A recent UK parliament POSTnote,[5] published in July 2021, highlighted how in particular young adults, women, those from minority ethnic communities, and people experiencing socio-economic disadvantage, were at increased risk of adverse mental health outcomes as a consequence of lockdown measures.

One of the core groups most affected in terms of wellbeing by the pandemic measures was families with a child under the age of five, particularly those families supporting any disabilities or further educational needs. Although some families were lucky enough to experience lockdowns as having a positive impact on their living circumstances,[8] multiple studies have now shown increases in anxiety, depression and other mental health issues in many young families.[9] And by default, these effects on pregnant women and new parents rippled out; caught in the crossfire were family members unable to meet and support the care of a new baby, and the midwives, health visitors and other healthcare professionals and volunteers who were unable to care for families in the way they valued and were so used to.

The pandemic and the first 1001 days

Pregnancy and the postnatal period are established as critical times in terms of health and wellbeing. Indeed, the 'first 1001 days' covering pregnancy and the first two years of life are now recognised by the government as a key time for investment and support, which can pay dividends in the long term.[10] Experiences during this time can affect a baby's cognitive, emotional and physical development, and have a lasting effect on the physical and emotional health of women and families.[11] Emphasis is placed on supporting new parents with issues including maternal physical recovery, infant feeding, infant care, and mental health.[12]

Strategies such as NHS England's 'Better Births' and the Maternity Transformation Programme seek to ensure that women receive personalised, kind, and woman-centred care throughout the perinatal period.[13] At the heart of this is knowledge of the importance of care that supports both physical and emotional health, along with recognition that treating women with dignity and respect is vital. Relationship-building is also key, with a focus on just how much difference continuity of care from the same health professionals can make. Developing a positive, supportive and respectful relationship during pregnancy has been shown to improve numerous birth and postnatal outcomes.[14]

Based on this knowledge, we have established programmes of antenatal, birth and postnatal care that seek to support mothers, babies and new families through this important period. We have copious evidence about what works best and what good care looks like (not that it always happens perfectly, far from it – but you know... the knowledge is there). However, during the first lockdown in March 2020, much of this care seemingly disappeared almost overnight. While some of it was reinstated, albeit often in an altered form, other elements are still not back to what they were even 18 months on. Subsequent lockdowns (and odd variations between countries and even local regions) meant that many pregnant and new families experienced a confusing and chaotic ride through maternity services and postnatal care.

The scale of the changes to maternity care, and their impact, was soon recognised. During the first lockdown the charity Birthrights raised the alarm over just how many families were contacting them about ways in which their pregnancy, birth and postnatal care was being affected.[15] Some of the changes included:

- Women having to be alone for scans and other appointments
- Partners not being allowed into the hospital until the mother was in established labour
- Partners being sent home straight after the birth
- Doulas not being allowed at the birth (or a forced choice between partner and doula)
- Restrictions on water births
- Restrictions on home births
- Restrictions on maternal requests for caesarean section
- No visitors on the postnatal ward
- Restrictions on 'visiting' babies in neonatal care
- Mask wearing during birth or postnatal care

These changes did not just occur in the UK. One research study that documented changes put in place across 32 countries in Europe found significant differences in the way that countries interpreted and applied guidance from the World Health

Organization in relation to delivering maternity care during the pandemic.[16] Overall, the paper highlighted:

- **All countries had some limitations on partners attending antenatal appointments, scans and during labour, although there were significant variations between countries.**
- **Protocols around breastfeeding differed significantly, including whether or not the woman should wear a mask during feeding, whether symptomatic women could breastfeed directly and how support was given.**
- **Separation of mother and baby if either tested positive differed between countries.**
- **Visiting to the neonatal unit varied between countries, with many even restricting the mother's access to 'visit' her baby.**
- **Regulations on mask-wearing differed between countries. In some countries all women had to wear them, in others partners had to wear them, and in others the mother only had to wear a mask if she had tested positive.**

Why did these changes occur? Ultimately it was a 'perfect storm': pressure on healthcare services due to the pandemic, a knock-on effect of reductions in social contacts that were deemed 'not necessary', and underlying anxieties about the potential impact of the virus on the health of pregnant women and their babies. At the start of the pandemic, we had little data about whether pregnant women would be at a greater risk of contracting the virus or experiencing significant side-effects. In previous viral outbreaks an increased risk had been seen due to immunological and cardiac changes in pregnancy making women more susceptible.[17] Protecting pregnant women should therefore have been a priority. But surely we also knew that high-quality antenatal, birth and postnatal care was vital to maternal and infant health outcomes? It appeared in some cases that this side of the story was forgotten.

It also appeared that more than ever women were falling foul of the 'precautionary principle' – the idea that it is 'better to be safe than sorry' that can pervade maternity services.[18] On the one hand you can understand the logic: we of course all want as many healthy babies (and mothers) as possible, so reducing as many risks as possible is common sense. But on the other hand, maternal wellbeing (both physical and psychological) is sometimes thrown under the bus as a result. There is always a balance to be struck, based on families' situations and preferences, with input from health professionals. But during Covid-19 we saw an almost knee-jerk reassertion of the most stringent 'precautionary' measures.

Having their maternity care and support suddenly cancelled or changed, and their birth plans curtailed, obviously had a significant impact on new families.[19] At the time of writing, in September 2021, we have toddlers whose whole lives have been lived through pandemic restrictions. Many have never been to a baby group or class, never properly met extended family, or even in some cases never interacted with another baby. And their parents have lived through these intensive months without ever having the benefits of a full support network to meet up with, cuddle or care for their baby. We'll look at the impact of this in more detail throughout the book, but to introduce the key points one interview study with new mothers in England highlighted what many of them were feeling or experiencing. They reported:

- A loss of the typical pregnancy experience including common milestones
- Anxiety due to little face-to-face contact with health professionals
- A loss of being able to share the experience with other new parents
- Concerns that phone appointments missed physical symptoms and warning signs
- Worries about their babies missing out on opportunities to socialise

- Few opportunities to seek reassurance from family and friends
- Partners missing out and feeling excluded leading to relationship tensions
- Fear about attending appointments on their own in case anything was wrong
- Increasing anxiety due to the frequency of changes to rules
- Loneliness and isolation at a time when contact was desperately needed
- Feeling abandoned by removal of choices and care

This book looks closely at what happened to parents and their babies (and those whose role it was to care for them) during the pandemic, and why. Perhaps most importantly, what can we learn and what can we do now to help repair the damage caused?

Note – if you're a new parent struggling to come to terms with everything that you've faced, you'll find a practical section especially for you at the end of this book.

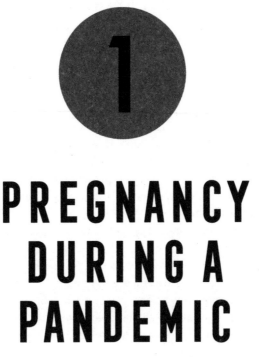

PREGNANCY DURING A PANDEMIC

PREGNANCY DURING A PANDEMIC

THE IMPACT UPON PHYSICAL AND MENTAL HEALTH

Experiences of pregnancy have been seriously affected by the pandemic. Expectant parents were faced with two main fears: would the virus affect the health and wellbeing of pregnant women and babies? And how would lockdowns and social distancing affect antenatal care? Understandably anxieties ran high, not helped by the media presenting manipulative and confusing messages about the risks during pregnancy and how care might be affected.

We now know that pregnant women as a group are at increased risk of complications if they become unwell with Covid-19. Protecting them and those who care for them was and still is important. However, as we will see in more detail later, there is a big difference between being at 'increased risk', and 'definitive harm' being caused to all pregnant women. Arguably the individual risk or likelihood of being seriously affected in terms of physical health was actually relatively low for many women without underlying health issues, but the negative psychological impact of changes to care was almost universal. And that's before we even consider the harm of fear-based messaging in the media that led some families to feel very unsafe indeed. There is a fine balance between protecting pregnant women and babies from the virus, and ensuring they receive the high-quality antenatal care we touched on in the introduction. Unfortunately, throughout the pandemic the balance has often been off.

What are the physical risks of Covid for pregnant women?

The evidence about whether pregnant women are at greater physical risk has changed over time. During the period when we were first going into lockdown, in March 2020, messaging was chaotic. There was a lack of data about the specific impact of Covid-19, but we knew from previous outbreaks of similar viruses, such as SARS (severe acute respiratory syndrome) and MERS (Middle East respiratory syndrome), that pregnant women, especially those in the third trimester, might be at increased risk due to alterations in immune system and cardiovascular function during pregnancy.[1] On the one hand there was talk of pregnant women needing to 'shield' (remain at home, avoiding all contact with others). And on the other hand we had guidance from the Royal College of Obstetricians and Gynaecologists (RCOG) published in late March 2020, which raised awareness of the potential risk of increased susceptibility but noted that at the time of publication there had been no cases of pregnant women dying from the disease.[2]

Of course, over time the number of infections increased and we sadly did have cases of pregnant women becoming very seriously unwell and dying of the virus. It is really difficult to try and track and measure outcomes for a disease that has only relatively recently emerged and is still ongoing, especially at the start of a pandemic when case numbers are relatively low. For research studies to have sufficient numbers to be statistically accurate, you need sufficient numbers of pregnant women experiencing the illness and complications. Therefore at the start of the pandemic we desperately needed data, but had to rely on case studies, as many pregnant women were (thankfully!) protected from catching the virus due to the lockdown.

But science doesn't ever (or rather shouldn't ever) base conclusions and policies on just one study, or even several, especially not case studies of individual women. It is the broader picture of research studies (taking into account how they were done and who was involved, and all the inevitable limitations) and how they fit together that should inform our decisions. Unfortunately, however, the news media searched for and manipulated anything they could spin to create more fear, in turn exacerbating the confusion around whether pregnant women were more at risk from the virus and its complications. A 'breaking news story' of a pregnant woman seriously ill or dying from Covid-19 infection is *of course* devastating, but it is not necessarily an indication that all pregnant women are at high risk. In reality, journalists and reporters know this, but it was disregarded in the pursuit of media market share.

Data soon began to accumulate that confirmed that although pregnant women were not at greater risk of developing Covid-19 infection in the first place, if they did catch the virus they were at risk of more serious complications as a result of the illness,[3] particularly during their third trimester.[4] Although most pregnant women who contracted Covid-19 only had mild symptoms (that probably didn't feel very mild, particularly in later pregnancy), some pregnant women did sadly die as a result of the virus due to complications exacerbated by the immune and cardiovascular changes of pregnancy. However, notably this direct impact of the infection was not the only cause of some maternal deaths.

In the UK data on maternal mortality rates are published in the MBRRACE (Mothers and Babies: Reducing Risk through Audits and Confidential Enquiries) report.[5] Two reports have been published since the start of the pandemic, examining maternal deaths as a consequence of Covid-19. The first was a rapid review examining deaths from 1 March–31 May 2020. It included the deaths of 10 women who died with Covid-19. Seven deaths were directly due to the virus (six from cardio-respiratory disease and one from a blood clot in the brain). Two deaths were from unrelated causes, but the women were infected with Covid-19. Data for one woman was unclear as no post-mortem had been carried out, but her death was thought to be due to Covid-19. All were in the last trimester of pregnancy when they became infected. Ninety per cent were from Black, Asian and minority ethnic (BAME) groups including Black (30%), Asian (50%) and Chinese (10%) backgrounds. For context, during the same period six pregnant or postnatal women died from other common causes of maternal death, including four from suicide and two from domestic abuse.

At the end of the first report the authors noted that '*It is reassuring that pregnant and postpartum women do not appear to be at higher risk of severe Covid-19 than non-pregnant women*'. However, in a second report including data from June 2020–March 2021 it was noted that the second wave of the virus brought a higher rate of infection and new variants of concern.[6] With more virus circulating, and therefore more likelihood of coming into contact with it, the data started to show that pregnant women were at a greater risk of Covid complications than non-pregnant women of reproductive age. It is important to remember that the overall individual risk, particularly to those without significant health complications, was still relatively low – but it had increased.

Overall, the second MBRRACE report identified 17 women who had died as a consequence of Covid-19 in the UK. To put these figures in the context of absolute risk, during the 10-month period that the report covers, approximately 587,700 women gave birth in the UK, giving an estimated maternal mortality rate of 2.4 in 100,000 births. It should be noted that this risk applies across all pregnant women whether they caught Covid-19 or not, and is not the risk of mortality if unwell with the virus. Also, the authors caution that MBRRACE maternal mortality estimations are usually based on figures over a three-year period to allow for any natural variations, so these data are not directly comparable. But for context there are approximately 70 maternal deaths during pregnancy or in the first six weeks postpartum every year in the UK. This data also gives averaged figures across all mothers. Risk for mothers from BAME groups, as we shall see below, is higher.

Ten of the seventeen women died from causes directly related to Covid-19, including cardio-respiratory complications (n=9) and thrombotic complications (n=1). Four women were positive for Covid at the time of their death but died from unrelated causes. However, three women were deemed to have died as a result of altered care, or engagement with care, due to the pandemic. For example, one woman was admitted to hospital with Covid-19. Her symptoms (e.g. fever) were believed to be due to Covid and she was placed in a bed and not observed for another 6.5 hours. It turned out that although she was infected with Covid, she had actually experienced a missed miscarriage and died from sepsis due to an intrauterine infection. Her symptoms of sepsis were overlooked due to the focus on the symptoms and diagnosis of Covid-19 infection.

The report examined the care the 10 women who died directly from their Covid infection received. Just one woman was considered to have received good care. Two were considered to have received care that could have been improved, but was unlikely to have prevented their death. However, for seven women improvements could have been made to their care which could have led to a 'difference in outcome', or in other words quite possibly have saved their lives.

Of the 10 women who died as a direct result of Covid infection, half were in their third trimester. In terms of risk factors 80% were overweight or obese, 60% were from Black, Asian and minority ethnic groups and 50% had a pre-existing mental health condition. However, no woman had a pre-existing physical health condition such as diabetes, hypertension or cardiac disease. It is unclear from the report how many pregnant women overall who gave birth during the report period were from BAME groups. Given that BAME groups make up approximately 13% of the UK population and approximately 587,000 women gave birth, we could assume that around 82,000 BAME women gave birth during that period. If six women died directly of Covid-19, this gives a rate of death of 7.3 in 100,000. Conversely, if four White women died directly of Covid-19 this gives a rate of death of 0.8 in 100,000, a shocking difference in the maternal death rate by ethnic group.

Please note that these are my estimates and are not directly taken from the MBRRACE report. However, the difference in death rate is clear and we will come back to this later.

In terms of hospital admissions for Covid-19 among pregnant women, a national population-based survey including all 194 obstetric units in the UK collected data on admissions and outcomes.[7] During a six-week period at the start of the pandemic, 427 pregnant women were admitted to hospital, which represented around 4.9 in every 1,000 women who gave birth during that period. Again, that figure is based on all births and not just those who had Covid-19. Additionally, the authors note that not all were seriously unwell; an increased cautionary tendency to admit pregnant women who were unwell may have inflated these figures. Most women who were admitted (81%) were in their third trimester – a figure that has been supported in other studies.[8]

In terms of who was admitted, 69% were overweight or obese, and 34% had pre-existing conditions such as diabetes or cardiac disease. Obese and overweight pregnant women have been more likely to be admitted to hospital with Covid-19 during pregnancy across many studies, as have those who are overweight or obese in the general population. It is likely that the association of obesity with other chronic illnesses, insulin resistance and inflammation, plays a role in exacerbating the impact of the virus.[9]

Additionally, as with the previous study, those from BAME groups were overrepresented. Here 56% were from BAME groups when BAME groups make up 13% of the general population in the UK. This can partly be explained by physiological factors. Pregnant women from BAME groups are more likely to have genetic risk factors or health comorbidities that place them at increased risk from viruses such as Covid-19. Other contributors include being more likely to live in densely populated or deprived areas where infection risk is higher.[10]

However, a crucial factor highlighted in many commentaries is the structural and institutional racism that places individuals at greater risk of health complications.[11] It is now established that women from BAME groups are at a greater risk of complications in the perinatal period even when we are not experiencing a global pandemic.[12] Increasingly research shows that women from BAME groups do not access the same level of support from health services during the antenatal and postnatal periods. This isn't due to a lack of awareness of services or their potential benefits, but rather due to racial inequalities in the suitability and accessibility of services currently offered, which mean that women avoid care or miss out on being cared for. Research has highlighted how a lack of cultural sensitivity, overt and covert issues of racism and a perceived lack of focus on individual needs can lead to vastly different care experiences.[13] Urgent reviews into this issue, specifically in relation to Covid-19, are needed to ensure equity in care.

Admission into hospital is not the same as admission into critical care. In the hospital admission study above 10% of women admitted to hospital needed critical care (n=41).[7] This represents a critical care rate of 1 in 2,400 women who gave birth during that period (i.e. across the population, not across those who were infected). All these women needed respiratory support, but just one woman was intubated. Sadly, 1% of hospitalised women died, this represents 1 in 18,000 women who gave birth during that six-week period. When this was examined according to the admission and mortality rates *at the time*, no difference in risk of critical care admission or death was seen between pregnant women with Covid-19 infection and rates in the general population of women of reproductive age. Of course every death is devastating to a family, especially when it seems that the death may have been preventable. But keeping this in context, in terms of the extent to which pregnant women 'needed' to be anxious, is important due to the effect of anxiety on other health-seeking behaviour. Hold this thought as we'll return to it in more detail later in this chapter.

The previous study was based on data from early on in the pandemic (1 March–14 April 2020) when cases and transmission were relatively low. More globally, a review paper updated in September 2020 analysed data from 192 studies including 67,271 women who attended or were admitted to hospital for any reason, including confirmed or suspected Covid-19 infection. This included research from numerous studies, predominantly conducted in the USA, China, Italy, Spain, Turkey, India and the UK. The overall rate of Covid-19 infection in women was 10% of pregnancies. This included a rate of 7% in studies where all women attending a hospital for any appointment or to give birth were tested and 28% when only women with symptoms were tested.[8] Overall, 3.3% were admitted to ICU, 1.5% needed ventilation and 0.8% died.

When you read these stats it's important to note that the researchers did not separate outcomes for Covid-19 from all other conditions. Therefore, these figures aren't necessarily due to Covid-19, and you have to consider what the 'normal' rate of these complications would be. This is tricky when you have a study which pools data from different countries, as different countries have different mortality and morbidity rates. Additionally, many studies included testing of women who attended a hospital because they were unwell, but would likely have missed those with mild symptoms (or who were asymptomatic) as they would not have attended. Therefore these data have to be considered in terms of 'women who we knew were positive for Covid-19' rather than '*all* women who tested positive for Covid-19'. Research has shown that the more severe the Covid-19 infection, the greater the risk of complications for a pregnant woman, and vice versa.[14]

Other studies have specifically compared outcomes for pregnant women with and without Covid-19. For example, one study in the US examined outcomes for 869,079 women giving birth across 499 medical centres between 1 March 2020 and 28 February 2021 (allowing for a much longer period of transmission and cases to occur). This included 18,715 who were infected with Covid-19 at the time of birth (approximately 2%). Women with Covid-19 had significantly higher rates of ICU admission (5.2 versus 0.9%), intubation or mechanical ventilation (1.5 versus 0.1%) and death (0.1 versus 0.01%). These data show that pregnant women were indeed at an increased risk of complications and mortality from Covid-19, but also statistically, at an individual level, that risk was not definitive. For example, even if 5% of women with Covid-19 are admitted to intensive care, 95% are not.[15] As an aside, the findings also raise serious questions about why pregnant women were not prioritised for vaccination and we will consider that in depth in Chapter 9.

What about babies?

Remarkably, the impact on babies in terms of Covid-19 infection has always been small. Review papers have now shown that the majority of babies born to mothers with a positive infection across multiple studies have themselves not tested positive.[16] There have now been multiple case studies of babies having no positive infection but having Covid-19 antibodies in their umbilical cord blood.[17] When babies have been infected with Covid-19 their symptoms have mostly been mild.[18]

For example, in the UK study above examining maternal admission to hospital with Covid-19 infection, the majority of infants remained well.[7] In terms of Covid infection, just 5% of babies tested positive, half of them within the first 12 hours after birth. It is possible that transmission occurred during pregnancy, but as the authors note, this was a large records-based study and no data was collected on circumstances around birth. It is possible that those babies contracted Covid during birth *or* from postnatal care.

In this study, half of babies with positive tests were admitted to the Neonatal Intensive Care Unit (NICU) compared to around 10% of all babies born to mothers without Covid-19.[7] Comparatively, in the global review paper looking at babies born to infected mothers, 28.1% were admitted to NICU.[8] For context, in the UK and USA 10–15% of babies are admitted to NICU each year, which suggests a higher rate of admission. However, the authors note that it is unclear why babies were admitted, and it could be (and most likely was) precautionary in many cases. In part it may also be due to an increase in premature births among pregnant women with Covid-19 (often for maternal not infant reasons).

Premature births

As with maternal mortality and hospitalisation rates, when we look at outcomes for babies during Covid-19, such as premature or stillbirths, it's important to consider what question is being studied. Some papers look at risk to babies when their mother is infected, while others look at rates across a hospital, large data set or even country. These papers obviously measure different things, i.e. the impact of a pregnant woman contracting the virus, versus the overall impact on the population of Covid-19 circulating. If pregnant women are avoiding social contacts and are at a relatively low overall risk of contracting the virus, the impact of the virus on pregnancy outcomes is going to be diluted across a large population.

In the UK study above that examined outcomes for mothers with the virus, around a quarter of women had a pre-term birth compared to a typical population rate of around 7–8%. However, it should be noted that the majority (80%) of these births were via elective caesarean or being induced rather than mothers going into pre-term labour. Half were induced due to maternal infection, i.e. because the mother was unwell, rather than issues with the baby. In the global review paper of babies born to infected mothers, 14.9% were born prematurely compared to an approximate global rate of 10%.[19]

In research studies that have looked at the impact across a country or hospital regardless of infection status, some studies have found a *reduction* in premature births. For example, a study in Denmark found a reduction in the rate of extremely premature births during March and April 2020 compared to these months in previous years.[20] Similar findings were seen for premature infants born at 32–36 weeks' gestation in the Lazio region of Italy.[21] However, a similar study in Sweden did not find any reduction.[22]

Overall, it appears that mothers who are infected with Covid-19 may be at increased risk of premature birth, both in terms of a decision being made to deliver their baby early, and a small increased risk of going into preterm labour. However, across populations, i.e. including those who were not infected, the risk appears to have reduced. This has been attributed to lower stress among many pregnant women who were furloughed or working from home, in that they did not need to commute and spend long days in the office. Significant personal variations are likely here, however, and as we will see later, not all frontline staff were able to work from home, probably increasing their stress. The reduction in premature births has also been attributed to lower levels of air pollution during lockdown, the closure of schools, and increased hygiene measures.[23]

Stillbirth

The same caveats that apply to the data and the questions being studied when we look at premature birth also apply to stillbirth. In the UK study examining maternal admission to hospital with Covid-19 infection, five babies sadly died, including three babies who were stillborn and two neonatal deaths.[7] However, these are not above expected figures. Three babies died due to obstetric complications and pre-existing conditions (rather than from Covid-19). For the remaining two, who were both stillborn, the cause of death was uncertain, and it was unclear whether Covid infection played any role. However, outside of the pandemic, around half of all stillbirths remain unexplained.[24] Likewise, in the global review paper of babies born to infected mothers, 0.7% were stillborn and 0.4% died in the neonatal period.[8] Global stillbirth rates vary enormously between countries and therefore it is difficult to compare these rates. Around 1.3% of babies are stillborn globally, the majority in the poorest regions in the world. Therefore Covid-19 infection itself does not appear to increase the stillbirth rate.

Looking at stillbirth rates across different countries, the evidence is mixed. Data from Sweden,[22] Canada,[25] and the US state of Philadelphia[26] reported no difference in stillbirth rates.

However, a study in the UK, based on a smaller sample from one London hospital, found an increased stillbirth rate in the early months of the pandemic (9.31 per 1,000 births) compared to before the pandemic (2.38 per 1,000 births). Notably no mother who experienced a stillbirth was infected or showing signs of Covid-19.[27] Similar increases were seen in an Italian study examining birth outcomes in the region of Lazio. Here stillbirth figures were three times higher in March–May 2020 than they were during the same months in previous years. Again Covid-19 infection did not appear to explain this.[21]

In many developing regions, an increase was also seen. In Nepal stillbirths increased from 14 in 1,000 births pre-pandemic to 21 in 1,000 births during it, alongside an increase in infant mortality rates from 13 per 1,000 births to 40 in 1,000 births.[28] In India intrauterine or stillbirth deaths increased from 2.25% to 3.15%.[29] No distinction was made between deaths potentially due to maternal Covid-19 infection and others.

Researchers have hypothesised about why stillbirths may have increased from a physiological perspective. One study examined 'placental pathology' during the pandemic – in other words, were placentas as healthy during the pandemic as they were before? Across their sample they found a significantly increased rate of abnormal placental perfusion (how well blood flows through the placenta carrying nutrients and oxygen) during the pandemic, which they thought might impact on the health and development of the baby in the womb. However, it should be noted that they did not see any change in stillbirth rates in their sample, although as their sample was based on one hospital, stillbirth numbers within the study would have been expected to be very low.[30]

A case study also reported on changes to the placenta, documenting a condition called villitis of the placenta in a mother with Covid-19. Villitis refers to inflammation of the chorionic villi, which are the structures covering the surface of the placenta that help deliver nutrients and oxygen to the baby. The researchers concluded that the mother's antiviral immune response (to Covid-19) led to the inflammation in the placenta, reducing how well the placenta worked.[31] Other cases studies have identified lesions on the placenta in women with Covid-19, which again affect how well the placenta can support the baby.[32]

Given that many of these studies reported no or low infection rates among mothers whose babies were stillborn, why might stillbirth rates be increasing if not directly due to infection? One explanation is reduced antenatal care attendance due to anxieties about seeking care during a pandemic. For example, in a study in the UK, attendance at an obstetric unit for concerns about reduced foetal movement dropped from an average of 22% of all pregnancies in the year before the pandemic to 18% in the first two months of lockdown.[33]

Likewise, in the studies in Nepal and India above,[28,29] the increase in stillbirth was attributed to a decrease in the number of mothers attending hospitals to give birth. In developing regions receiving antenatal care and giving birth in a healthcare facility with a skilled birth attendant is especially important in reducing maternal and infant mortality. In the Swedish study, where no change in the rate of stillbirth was found, the authors noted that there was no reduction in maternal healthcare visits, hypothesising that perhaps the fewer lockdown measures in Sweden at the time meant that women were not discouraged from seeking care, as may have occurred in other countries with more restrictions.[22]

The impact of anxiety, risk messaging and fearmongering on pregnant women's wellbeing and decision-making

In the UK it appears that we ended up in a situation where messaging that was supposed to reduce the spread of Covid-19 ended up scaring some women so much that they avoided seeking care that was actually needed. We also saw this in other areas of health, not just maternity. One study tracking attendance at accident and emergency departments in London during the early months of the pandemic recorded a 50% reduction.[34] In part this could genuinely be due to fewer accidents, perhaps as a result of fewer car journeys and lowered stress (for some). But that does not explain the extent of the reduction. People were staying away because they were scared of contracting the virus, and worried about the pressure that the health service was under. Although we have an issue of over-attendance at such centres in normal times, these figures show that some people were staying away when they actually needed care because they were disproportionately scared of the virus. The same appears to be true when we examine the research into women's experiences of pregnancy.

An ongoing issue central to public health messaging is how we communicate levels of risk.[35] There are numerous different ways we can do this, helpful and otherwise, but some appear to be preferred by the media in terms of their ability to stir up fear and panic.

1. What is the risk to us as a population as a whole?

One way of looking at risk is to consider what proportion of a population you might expect to become infected and become seriously unwell. How many people might we see die or develop long-term health problems due to Covid-19 across our whole population? This is a figure often used by the government, health boards and other public health services because they have to consider the implications for the population as a whole. If you are 'responsible' for delivering healthcare to a population of 66 million, you need to be thinking about the sum of all the treatment and other impacts of an increased proportion of them (no matter how small) becoming unwell or dying.

This is an important figure as obviously we would prefer it if preventable deaths and disabilities were avoided. But it also matters in terms of the impact on our health services and economy. If you have one million people seriously ill and needing care then that affects the healthcare system, which isn't set up to cope with so many additional patients. It also costs money and resources in terms of medical supplies, hospital space and staff to treat them. These beds, resources and money get taken away from other less urgent healthcare issues – hence the knock-on impact we've seen due to operations and other healthcare being cancelled. This is especially problematic if you live in a country where the government has been systematically disinvesting in and demolishing the healthcare system that so many rely on.

2. What is the risk to us as individuals?

Additionally, we have data about what our *individual* risk is. We might care very much about how many of the population might get unwell, but what does that actually mean for us on an individual level? Just how concerned should we be? Reading headlines about the numbers of infections and deaths can be terrifying, and is actually also ineffective at improving health outcomes. Although some would argue that fear-based messages are designed to get people to wake up and take notice, this technique has been shown not to work, as if you scare people too much they start to ignore you or act even more recklessly.[36] Instead, context and accuracy are vitally important. If we don't have any context for our individual risk, or indeed what the infections and deaths figures mean in context (for example, around 2,000 people die every day in the UK from other health issues and accidents),[37] then how can we make a sensible judgement (and take sensible precautions)?

There are two ways that our individual risk can be expressed. Firstly, you have something called 'absolute risk', which is *the chance of something happening to you*. So if, for example, you assume that all people are at equal risk, the population is 60 million people and you expect 60,000 people to die, your absolute risk of dying is 0.1% (or in other words, a 99.9% chance of not dying). This isn't an accurate figure – just a nice neat mathematical example to illustrate the point.

In terms of more accurate data, as I write approximately 10% of the UK population has tested positive for Covid-19 infection (via lab-reported PCR test) since the start of the pandemic. In the US it is slightly higher at approximately 12%.[38] Even after all my research for this book, this figure is a bit surprising to me. With all the media headlines I expected that figure to be much higher – although presumably the actual figure *is* higher due to asymptomatic or missed cases (or avoidance of testing). And one in 10 people still constitutes a high proportion of people experiencing an illness and the associated consequences of time away from work, caring responsibilities and of course for the health service. This proportion would also have likely been much higher without containment methods. It's just that if you went by how some of the news media have portrayed the data, you would have thought people who hadn't been infected were as rare as hen's teeth right now, when in fact 90% of us haven't been infected (or haven't realised we have been).

Of those who have been infected, approximately 8% have been hospitalised and there have been approximately 130,000 deaths, giving a case fatality rate (the proportion of people who have the disease who die) of 1.9%, and an overall population mortality rate of roughly 0.2%.[38] There are limitations with the data (as there are with any data), including missed positive cases due to people being asymptomatic or not testing, and people dying 'with' Covid-19 and not directly because of it, which may mean that the actual death rate may be slightly lower.

Looking at this with a cold statistical hat on it translates to a relatively low individual risk percentage wise – although clearly one that carries a devastating impact for families who are affected. Although the mortality rate from Covid is much lower[37] compared to deaths from other diseases such as dementia,

Alzheimer's disease, cancer and heart disease, the suddenness and novelty of the virus, its immediacy, and the fact that it felt like an avoidable disease made the risk of this illness feel greater for many people. As noted previously, it is also a major problem for public health services if you have six million people with a virus and over 500,000 of them need hospital care. This also has a knock-on effect on non-urgent healthcare, contributing to the huge waiting lists we discussed in the introduction.

However, we also know that not everyone has an equal chance of dying from the virus. We knew early on that underlying health factors and older age in particular increased the risk of someone dying or becoming seriously ill (with age being the predominant risk factor, often crossing over with underlying health issues – while diabetes was a risk factor, for example, an 85-year-old with diabetes had a much higher risk than a 35-year-old with diabetes). We knew that some of the mortality data was affected by older people dying of other causes – 'with' rather than 'from' the virus. In many cases the virus caused the death of someone who was much older and in poor health. It is likely to have caused many 'earlier' deaths as opposed to 'early' deaths. This is of course still devastating for individual families, and for us as a society, especially given the feeling that deaths from the virus could have been avoided and families had their time together cut short. There were many situations (such as sending Covid-positive patients from hospital to nursing homes) where this could likely have been reduced.

However, when it comes to balancing how anxious a younger pregnant woman or new parent needed to be about themselves or their baby, messaging should clearly have placed this in context. As we will see later in the chapter, anxiety among some pregnant women about catching the virus was so high that they avoided antenatal care, with devastating consequences. But the data that was typically trotted out in the press about a '2% mortality rate' did not apply to the majority of those pregnant or with a new baby (recognising the raised risk of some groups discussed earlier such as for underlying health conditions and ethnicity). You cannot transfer a mortality rate that is heavily skewed towards much older people (the median age of death has typically remained above 80 throughout the pandemic[39]) to a younger person whose individual risk is much lower. As we saw earlier, the approximate mortality rate for infected pregnant women was around 0.1%[15] or 1 in 18,000 of all pregnant women.[7] Still serious, absolutely. But a lot less than 2%. Accurate and contextualised data, rather than broad statistics, is an important part of informed decision-making.

Of course, there were also concerns about how the virus might affect a growing or new baby (which, as we have seen, thankfully turned out to be mostly unfounded). And becoming ill is never fun during pregnancy or when caring for a new baby (even if technically the illness is 'mild'). There were also concerns about how long symptoms and post-viral illness could last. And although the individual risk for many was low, it was certainly not zero, and across our large population some healthy individuals were seriously affected. Altogether it was a worrying time for anyone who was pregnant or caring for a new baby – but risk should nonetheless have been sensitively communicated and balanced against the evidence-based need for antenatal and postnatal care (including emotional support and social contact).

So where did high levels of anxiety come from? Most likely from skewed perceptions of individual risk, which were heightened by media reporting. We recognised that many groups in our population *were* at higher risk, and that the impact across our population in terms of the tragedy of avoidable deaths, the impact on the healthcare system and economic damage could be huge. How do you stop that? Well, we knew the virus spread through human contact and that until vaccines were in place (and successful, and uptake high), the only way to reduce the spread of the virus was to reduce contacts between humans.

Unfortunately, that also had untold negative consequences for those affected by the regulations put in place. It was particularly hard for many at low health risk but who felt the economic, work and social consequences more severely. This is where fear messaging and anxiety took hold. The government needed to persuade those at low individual risk to follow guidelines which felt detrimental to their personal situations. Data and graphs were used to hammer home the point, with the consequence that personal anxiety was most likely increased and exacerbated for some. Rather than understanding the logic for precautions, and being able to situate their own individual risk within this, some interpreted the risk of contracting Covid as catastrophic, taking measures that may ultimately have done more harm than good. The media jumped on the opportunity to terrify people because fear sells (or at least makes them money in online advertising). And pregnant women were caught up in it all.

From the data earlier in this chapter we can see that pregnant women, particularly those with underlying risk factors, were at statistically increased risk of serious complications from Covid-19, which is why additional care and support was needed. But risk from Covid-19 was only ever meant to be one part of the story. We know that antenatal care during pregnancy can be lifesaving for both mother and baby in helping spot complications before they get more serious, or providing the opportunity to intervene. It also supports maternal mental health, helps support a healthy pregnancy (e.g. by supporting decisions around alcohol consumption and smoking) and most importantly is valued by women. Although in the UK we have become used to a relatively low risk of maternal and infant mortality and morbidity, antenatal care is one of the core reasons why these are so low.[40] In the UK the programme of antenatal care includes initial and ongoing physical check-ups, blood tests and scans to monitor the health of both mother and baby.[41]

Unfortunately, the fear provoked by the pandemic media circus led to such high levels of anxiety among some pregnant women that their mental health and eventually care-seeking behaviour was affected. The risk of Covid-19 infection was real, but at an individual level the risk for those without risk factors was usually not so catastrophic that they needed to avoid doing things that would have helped support their health and wellbeing during pregnancy. And this is sadly what happened in some cases – things that were put in place or that some women ended up doing as a consequence of this fear quite possibly created more risk to them as individuals than Covid-19 itself.

We know that anxiety levels were high. For example, one study in Denmark found that many pregnant women were concerned that they were at very high risk from infection. In a survey of 255 pregnant women, 50% believed that their risk of getting infected during pregnancy was 'high', with 36% believing that if they got infected there was a high risk that they would be severely ill. In terms of worries about their baby, 39% believed that there was a high risk that their baby would be affected.[42]

During the first lockdown messaging at first was mixed (read chaotic) about whether pregnant women needed to shield or not.[43] Eventually pregnant women were advised to follow the social distancing guidance given to others, such as staying home as much as possible and social distancing. However, one interview study with pregnant women found that many felt they needed to take extra precautions such as washing shopping or quarantining post and other items.[44] Three women (10%) were shielding (e.g. not going out at all) because they believed that this was what pregnant women needed to do.

Others were worried about the risk of someone else coming into their household to care for an older child during labour. One woman described asking a family member who was planning to care for her older child to completely shield for two weeks before doing so in order to reduce risk for her newborn baby. When thinking about lockdown measures easing, many wanted to keep to social distancing and avoiding contacts, to reduce the risk of catching the virus while pregnant or because of fear about visitors passing it to their newborn. Many women felt significant stress and a psychological burden in trying to continually balance perceived measures for Covid-19 safety with behaviours that would support them in other ways, e.g. seeing a family member, or contacting a health professional.

This study wasn't an isolated example. In Australia, where Covid-19 infection rates have been relatively low compared to many countries, some pregnant women took more precautions than were advised, avoiding any public transport or meeting with others, even before any regulations were in place.[45] Again it was common for parents with older children to take them out of school in the weeks before the birth so that the chances of them catching the virus and needing to isolate (and therefore affecting birth plans) was reduced. Others were scared about extended family eventually meeting their baby, even when they could. Some were worried about older siblings touching the baby, discouraging contact.

Alongside high levels of generalised anxiety (which we know is distressing and may even be detrimental to babies during pregnancy – more on this in a moment), data also started to emerge that showed some women were avoiding what was most likely important care. In a survey of 81 obstetric units in the UK at the start of the pandemic units were asked whether they were experiencing any reduction in women turning up in emergency situations such as for bleeding or reduced foetal movement.[46] Overall, 86% reported that they were seeing fewer women, with 28% of units seeing a reduction in emergency attendance of over 50%.

It is unlikely that fewer women were experiencing unexplained bleeding or reduced foetal movement (or at least, not to that extent). So what was happening? Three things. First, pregnant women were scared of attending hospitals or accessing services due to their perceived risk of catching the virus. In a survey of 1,455 women who were pregnant or gave birth during the early weeks of the pandemic, many who needed to contact their midwife for issues such as reduced foetal movement felt reluctance or anxiety in doing so. Many felt that they needed to balance the risk of something being seriously wrong with the risk of Covid-19 exposure in hospital, and decided that the threat from Covid-19 was greater. Some did not even want to risk ringing their midwife for advice as they feared they would be made to go into hospital to be checked.

This fear also applied to routine appointments. One study found that some women were considering avoiding face-to-face appointments such as anomaly scans or blood tests as they felt they were too risky.[47] Another found that the more health anxiety women were experiencing around Covid-19, the more likely they were to cancel and avoid antenatal appointments.[48] It is notable that women could experience severe health anxiety about one threat (Covid-19), but not about another: the established risks of pregnancy that are reduced by antenatal care attendance. The rolling 24-hour news media and constant reminders of the Covid threat are most likely responsible for this.

Secondly, the studies above found that women had heard so many stories about healthcare systems being overwhelmed that they did not want to put pressure on midwives.[47] Some felt that their questions were not important enough in the grand scheme of the severity of Covid, and that healthcare professionals were only able to deal with emergency situations. Others felt embarrassed to seek support for issues they thought didn't matter compared to what they saw as the life-or-death importance of Covid.

Finally, pregnant women were also scared of catching the virus because they were worried that being Covid positive would impact their care during birth.[49] Women expressed concerns that they would receive different care, that staff would not want to look after them and that they would be forced to have a caesarean section rather than the birth they hoped for. Others were worried about what would happen to their baby after birth. Would they be separated? Would their baby catch the infection? Might they or their baby catch the infection from others on the ward? Women felt a huge stigma at the idea of testing positive, exacerbated by the idea that if you caught the virus it was because you had broken rules or did not wash your hands.

Women were also anxious about giving birth. In a study in Italy some women talked about being terrified about going into hospital to give birth because they believed that the risk of infection was so high.[50] Some were planning home births even when their pregnancies were not low risk because they believed the risk of Covid-19 infection was far greater than any obstetric complication. Many pregnant women in the UK felt the same.[49] What would happen when they went into hospital to give birth? Would they be exposed? Would staff have enough PPE and be safe? Would they need to wear a mask, and should they bring their own?

Sadly these fears were ultimately implicated in the deaths of several women in the UK. Four women in the MBRRACE report delayed or avoided care due to fear of infection. One woman developed a cough in late pregnancy but did not want to attend hospital due to fear of catching Covid-19. She died at home of the virus without having had any contact with healthcare professionals. Another woman had no antenatal care at all because she was concerned about catching the virus. She sadly died after giving birth alone at home. Two other women had symptoms of Covid-19 but did not want to be hospitalised and declined admission. They were both admitted critically unwell a few days later and died.[7]

On the other side of this story, however, was the lack of support for measures to reduce the risk for those who *were* in more high-risk situations. In terms of those in higher-risk frontline jobs, measures should have been taken to assess their risk. Even before the pandemic all pregnant women should have been given a risk assessment at work. The Department of Health and Social Care issued guidance that all pregnant employees should undergo an individual workplace safety assessment and, if the risk was deemed to be high, employers should consider how to redeploy them or enable them to work from home. Where adjustments were not possible due to the role or workplace, women should be suspended on paid leave.[51] However this clearly did not happen. A report from Pregnant Then Screwed in April 2020, including 490 pregnant NHS workers, found that 24% of those working for the NHS felt unsafe – with 31% of those from Black, Asian and minority ethnic groups feeling this way.[52] One reason for feeling unsafe was due to not being able to socially distance. Despite the guidance 25% of pregnant NHS workers could not do this in their role and nothing had been put in place to mitigate their risk.

This situation was echoed in another study. Among pregnant women who worked in NHS, social care or other frontline roles, almost half were concerned about staying safe. Many had been told that they had no choice but to remain in clinical patient-facing roles.[49] Others were facing not being paid. One woman in the early stages of pregnancy described how she currently wasn't being given any shifts in her job as a community care worker as it was deemed too risky, but she wasn't given sick pay so she had lost her income.[53] For some this had catastrophic consequences. In the MBRRACE report one pregnant woman with a BMI of over 50 (placing her at greater clinical risk) was returned to a frontline role in a care setting during the third trimester of her pregnancy. There was no record of a workplace safety assessment. She died from her infection.[7]

We also know that pregnant women from BAME groups were more likely to be placed at risk of infection, despite their increased personal risk. In general, people from BAME groups were more likely to work in frontline positions during the pandemic than those from White backgrounds.[54] In the UK 21% of NHS employees are from BAME backgrounds compared to BAME groups making up approximately 13% of the UK population. Furthermore, people from BAME groups are much more likely to work in frontline NHS roles compared to managerial or 'back office' roles.[55] Likewise in the US 43% of Black and Latino workers are employed in public-facing service jobs compared to 25% of White workers.[56]

Therefore, anxiety was naturally increased for women from BAME backgrounds as they knew that the data was showing an increased risk of serious complications. However, there appeared to be little information or reassurance about how women could be better supported. For example, in the *Babies in Lockdown* report (a survey of 5,474 pregnant women and new parents in the UK during the first lockdown), one mother expressed her fears about how the increased risk from Covid-19, plus the known increased maternal mortality rates among BAME women, was making her feel increasingly anxious.[57] And in another study two pregnant African-Caribbean women explained how they had been told by health professionals that they were more likely to die from Covid-19, but not why or what would happen to help protect them, leaving them understandably terrified.[49] Likewise, in another UK study a mother from a BAME background talked about how her older children were worried that when she went into hospital to give birth she would die as they'd seen so many stories around the risks of Covid-19.[53]

Anxiety, fear and mental health

Understandably, the combined impact of worrying about their own health, the health and safety of their baby and what birth in the time of Covid-19 would look like seriously affected the wellbeing of pregnant women.[58] One study in Italy at the start of the pandemic asked pregnant women in the later stages of pregnancy to describe how they were feeling about giving birth. The researchers asked them how they felt before the pandemic and how they now felt. The difference in how many felt different emotions before and during the pandemic was significant:

- Joy: 63% before and 17% now
- Safety: 38% before and 7% now
- Serenity: 25% before and 1% now
- Fear: 7% before and 49% now
- Anxiety: 2% before and 32% now
- Worry: 1% before and 19% now
- Loneliness: 1% before and 32% now
- Danger: 0% before and 19% now

Notably, when the researchers explored what pregnant women tended to be most scared about in terms of giving birth, fears before the pandemic were often about the pain of childbirth. However, during the pandemic women were more fearful about birth restrictions and loneliness during and after birth than they were about actually giving birth to their babies. Similar findings emerged in a UK study.[53] When pregnant women were asked how they were feeling, 'anxious' was one of the most commonly used words, with 90% feeling more anxious about giving birth during the pandemic than they had before. For some this was crippling. One woman described not being able to get out of bed or off the sofa as she was so paralysed with anxiety.

Another study in the US explored how many pregnant women were experiencing high levels of stress in the early months of the pandemic.[59] Over 4,000 women completed the 'Pandemic-Related Pregnancy Stress Scale' which was designed to measure two key types of stress: preparedness stress (feeling unprepared to give birth or care for a baby due to the pandemic) and perinatal infection stress (worries about herself or the baby getting infected). Overall, 27% reported high levels of preparedness stress and 29% high levels of perinatal infection stress. These two types of stress were linked but also distinct for some: 18% of women scored highly on both measures.

As with many studies exploring the impact of Covid-19, stress was related to wider stressful experiences. Mothers who were younger, single parents or in their first pregnancy had higher levels of stress. Likewise, those whose job or income had been affected by Covid suffered more. Complications during pregnancy including previous loss, multiple birth or underlying health conditions increased stress. Changes to antenatal care and birth plans were associated with higher stress due to uncertainty. Finally, women of colour had higher stress levels.

The irony here is that one of the things that we know reduces and helps prevent maternal stress during pregnancy is ... regular contact with health professionals. A strong midwife–mother relationship which is consistent, builds over time and has respect and trust at its heart helps support mothers' wellbeing during pregnancy. As we will see in the next chapter, this was one major aspect that was significantly affected as a result of Covid restrictions. Just when women needed that established connection the most, it was restricted or taken away.

Reflecting on specific Covid-19 related anxieties, an Italian study conducted in March 2020 (during the start of the Italian lockdown) explored the concerns of 178 pregnant women.[60] Overall, women were worried about the impact of catching the virus on growth restriction (65%), preterm birth (51%), and birth abnormalities (47%). In another study three-quarters of pregnant Chinese women were afraid of giving birth during the pandemic due to fears about how the virus might harm their baby.[61]

In terms of clinical measures of mental health, a meta-analysis of 23 studies exploring the impact of the pandemic on mental health during pregnancy found that rates of psychological distress were high. On average across the studies 37% of pregnant women had symptoms of anxiety, 31% symptoms of depression, 70% were experiencing psychological distress about the pandemic and 49% were experiencing insomnia.[62] Typically studies show a rate of antenatal anxiety or depression of somewhere around 10%.[63] Another study in California compared antenatal depression rates before and during the pandemic, finding an increase from

25% to 51%.[64]

The same picture has been painted in many different countries, including China,[65] Turkey,[66] Canada[67] and Japan.[68] While each country has different typical rates of antenatal depression, the same pattern emerged: women who were pregnant during the pandemic were displaying increased symptoms of depression. Further analyses of what was causing this all focussed broadly on the same three factors: fears about catching the virus itself, worries about social isolation and a lack of support, and changes to and reduction in antenatal care.

Why are these increased symptoms of anxiety and depression such an issue? Well first of all we obviously do not want women suffering with anxiety and depression, especially if these symptoms have been exacerbated disproportionately by media scaremongering. But secondly anxiety and depression can have longer-lasting effects. Anxiety and depression during pregnancy are risk factors for continued anxiety and depression after birth.[69] Additionally they have been associated with birth complications such as premature delivery and more interventions, with some studies finding an increased risk of growth restriction.[70] There is also some evidence that at very high levels anxiety can negatively affect infant health and development, by affecting immune, metabolic and endocrine pathways.[71]

So what's the key message of this chapter? Basically, it is vital that any model that estimates the impact of Covid-19 on a particular demographic group also takes into account the unintended or natural consequences of creating high levels of anxiety. For some women, the fear created around the virus will have had much more catastrophic unintended consequences for their health than the virus itself likely would have. We must ensure that risk-based messaging for pregnant women is accurate, personalised and put in the context of the importance of antenatal care for them and their baby.

2

HOW DID THE PANDEMIC AFFECT CARE DURING BIRTH?

HOW DID THE PANDEMIC
AFFECT CARE DURING BIRTH?

We've considered the impact of the messaging about the risk of the virus on women's mental health, anxiety and engagement with antenatal care. But this was not the only way in which women's antenatal care and support during their pregnancy and birth was affected. As we have learned, one of the main ways in which pregnant and birthing families were affected during the pandemic was in terms of changes to birth plans and choices, the intensity and perceived quality of care given, and their relationships with midwives and other professionals. The potential for a negative impact of this upon maternal and infant health and wellbeing is monumental, but of course again it appears to have been thought of as completely separate from the risks of the virus to pregnant women, and thus barely considered. What is the risk to a pregnant woman from Covid-19? And what is the risk to her from increased stress, a lack of continuity of care and increased intervention? The answer to those questions will be different for every family. But let's look more closely at why this matters, and how.

We have a wealth of evidence about the importance of supporting families through the perinatal period. We know that care during this time can have many physiological and psychological effects, and that these can be long lasting. Indeed, the World Health Organization recognises the importance of a 'positive pregnancy experience' in supporting mothers through birth and into motherhood.[1] Childbirth is a life-changing, transformative experience for many women, often seen as a rite of passage that many pregnant women simultaneously look forward to and are anxious about. Care received during pregnancy and birth is fundamental in how a woman experiences and remembers this important time.[2]

What does positive perinatal care look like? There are lots of different elements, many beyond the scope of this book, but here are some of the central pillars:

1. Care that promotes maternal wellbeing

We know that maternal stress during pregnancy, birth and the postnatal period not only affects maternal mental health, but can also have physiological impacts on a woman's pregnancy, birth and baby. Raised levels of stress hormones such as cortisol have been linked to an increased risk of preterm birth, birth complications and even foetal development.[3] Birthing environments that are focused on promoting trust, calm and safety are associated with better physiological and psychological birth outcomes. Conversely, high levels of tension and stress can slow down labour and increase the likelihood of interventions and complications.[4]

2. Care that is consistent

A Cochrane review of the evidence for continuous care emphasised its importance. Continuous support from midwives is associated with fewer birth interventions, reduced use of pain relief and shorter labours.[5] In addition, support from birth partners is valued by both mothers and partners, and leads to better birth and infant outcomes. Care from midwives and birth partners is typically complementary, with both providing care in different but overlapping ways.[6]

3. Care that centres women

Antenatal care that places women at its centre is based on a model of care in which the woman has control, can make her own choices and is involved in all aspects of her care.[7] Preferences should be respected. Communication should be clear. Women's autonomy and ability to make choices should be emphasised.[8] Research has revealed the importance of care that feels as though it is supporting both physical and emotional needs, with an emphasis on developing relationships between families and health professionals.[9] Ultimately care given should leave pregnant and birthing women feeling empowered.[10]

4. Care with informed decision-making and choice at its core

When women have the opportunity to make genuine informed decisions about their care during pregnancy and birth, and trust the health professionals around them to support them in this, they are more likely to describe their birth experience as positive, regardless of any complications that emerge.[11] The opportunity to reflect on and plan for preferred birth options in particular is associated with greater confidence going into birth and more positive feelings about birth during the postnatal period.[12] A central important aspect is having the opportunity to plan options that fit a family best, whether that be a home or hospital birth, a repeat caesarean or vaginal birth after caesarean and so on.

The NHS often talks about the importance of 'shared decision-making' between health professionals and women, but really the emphasis should be on 'family-centred decision making' and 'informed choice', where families receive sufficient information and support from their health professionals to make the decisions they feel work best for them. Shared decision-making during pregnancy and birth has been shown to help reduce maternal anxiety, improve decision-making and boost confidence in feeling that the best choice had been made.[13] It also helps strengthen relationships between families and health professionals.[14]

The right for women to receive this care is enshrined in policy.

For example the *National Maternity Review* (2019) emphasised that birth plans should be '*centred on the woman, her baby and her family, based around their needs and their decisions, where they have genuine choice, informed by unbiased information*'.[15] Many of these elements are at the heart of the NHS Maternity Transformation Programme and Better Births strategy.[16] The plan includes a commitment to ensure that:

1. All women have a personalised care plan
2. All women are able to make choices about their maternity care during pregnancy, birth and postnatally
3. Most women receive continuity of the person caring for them during pregnancy, birth and postnatally
4. More women are able to give birth in midwifery settings (at home and in midwifery units)

A recent qualitative systematic review exploring what mattered to women during pregnancy and birth highlighted aspects such as the following:[2]

- The support of a birth companion
- Continuity of care through pregnancy and birth
- Giving birth in an environment that feels safe and supportive
- Sensitive and kind care from staff
- Wanting to make informed decisions over birth preferences including interventions

Unfortunately we know that even outside the pandemic shared decision-making, informed choice and woman-centred care does not always happen due to pressures on health professionals' time, staffing issues and hospital policies and politics.[17] However, it seems that the pressures of the pandemic took everything we knew about what works well in supporting pregnant and birthing families and shoved it in a dark cupboard somewhere. All the benefits and risks of caring for women and their families in a certain way during pregnancy and birth appeared to be discarded during our efforts to reduce transmission of the virus.

What changes were made to care?

As we saw in the introduction, we knew from anecdotal experiences on social media and through contacts with organisations such as Birthrights that changes had rapidly been made to care in the early stages of the pandemic. These changes were highlighted in a survey of maternity services across the UK that documented what modifications to care had been made. Data was collected from 17 May–15 June 2020. In total 81 sites responded, representing 42% of 194 UK obstetric units.[18]

Overall, 70% of units reported a reduction in antenatal appointments. This included reductions in:

- **Obstetric appointments for high-risk women (28%)**
- **Maternal medicine appointments (22%)**
- **Foetal medicine appointments (25%)**
- **Specialist midwifery appointments (26%)**

For the way appointments were conducted, 89% reported conducting antenatal appointments remotely, including:

- **Telephone calls (88%)**
- **Video calls using widely available software (12%)**
- **Video calls using specially designed software (26%)**

In terms of modifications to the types of service offered, a reduction was seen in:

- **Screening services for foetal anomalies (15%)**
- **Change to in-home blood pressure monitoring (79%)**
- **Change to in-home urine testing for those with high blood**

pressure (32%)
- Screening pathways for gestational diabetes (a single blood test at 26–28 weeks (70%)
- Face-to-face appointments for gestational diabetes (88%)
- Growth scans for foetal monitoring (56%)
- Indicators for antenatal steroid (33%)

For birth options, a reduction was seen in:

- Availability of home birth or midwife-led unit (59%)
- Availability of water birth (32%)
- Caesareans without clinical indication (5%)
- Suspension of some indications for induction of labour (17%)

For postnatal care:
- Reduction in routine visits for low risk women (55%)
- Use of telephone or video call (57%)
- Increase in using students or care assistants to conduct appointments (11%)

What was the impact of these changes?

Many women experienced changes to their care, depending on what their birth plans were and their own individual pregnancy risks and needs.[19] Thinking more broadly about the impact of these changes first, many women, particularly those who were about to give birth at the start of the pandemic when everything was suddenly in flux, talked about the shock and anxiety they felt when they didn't know what to expect. They had spent the majority of their pregnancy planning for what they expected their options to be, for this to suddenly be whipped away from them at the last moment. Although birth often doesn't go exactly to plan, certain aspects were predictable before the pandemic, such as partners being allowed to stay during labour. Women found the media speculation around all of this particularly challenging.

Apart from the emotional impact of not being able to plan, women found the uncertainty and the frequently changing rules exhausting.[20] They described it as being in a state of 'problem-solving', which was challenging at the best of times, let alone when sleep-deprived, heavily pregnant or with a newborn. Women also talked about feeling 'cheated' out of appointments and anxious that things might have been missed. One woman described how at the start of her pregnancy her midwife had sat down and explained all the different appointments and their importance, only for them to suddenly be cancelled or replaced with phone calls. Mothers would understandably question whether these appointments were important in the first place, or whether they were not receiving important care they needed.[19]

The fear that symptoms would be missed was not unrealistic. In the MBBRACE report one woman contacted her GP because she was experiencing extreme back pain, but she did not tell them she was pregnant.[21] As it was a remote consultation her GP did not realise she was pregnant. She was prescribed analgesics. She died several days later due to sepsis. Another woman had a telephone consultation with a practice nurse at the peak of the second wave. She had a cough but somehow Covid-19 infection was not considered and she was diagnosed with a chest infection. She died from Covid-19 pneumonia the next day.

As time went on women became more resigned to the changes they would have to face. The emotional burden of preparing themselves for these changes and their impact was intense. In one interview study with women in Ireland participants talked about having to prepare themselves for things such as their partner not being present or being sent home straight after the birth, or needing to attend appointments for complications alone. This additional emotional load was intense, with women stoically talking about what they simply had to do.[22] Others talked about the grief and loss they were experiencing about the pregnancy, birth and newborn experience they realised they were never going to have.[23] Some had spent a long time dreaming about moments such as family or older children coming to the hospital to meet their baby, or being able to share the experience of a scan with their partner, and now everything had changed.

Some women found the way changes were communicated to them difficult to handle. Although many found that care was respectful, and midwives were supportive of the huge emotional impact of the changes, some women found communication very abrupt and not sensitive to their needs. The suggestion was that they simply needed to 'put up with it' and there was little point in complaining as this would not change things. This may have been true, but it doesn't mean that the loss and anxiety women were experiencing about their changed birth plans did not matter.[19] Others felt that there was simply a lack of recognition from some (including health professionals, friends and family and the public) of how the uncertainty around the pandemic and birth was anxiety-inducing.[24] Studies comparing satisfaction with care given during birth often showed a decrease for women giving birth during the pandemic.[25]

It is highly likely that all these changes had an impact on the higher rates of maternal anxiety and depression during pregnancy that we saw in the previous chapter (and the continued high rates during the postpartum period that we will consider in more detail in Chapter 7). In turn it is logical to assume that this heightened level of anxiety and stress through pregnancy and birth probably increased birth interventions and complications. As discussed earlier, we know that when birthing environments are calm and women feel as confident and supported as possible, birth is more likely to entail fewer complications.[4] High levels of stress hormones interfere with the progression of labour from a hormonal perspective, while women who are feeling highly anxious may find it more challenging to use psychological strategies to manage pain.[26]

Data from the UK, Ireland and the US has shown a slight rise in the number of caesarean sections.[27] However, variation was seen in this across the period of the pandemic and appeared to be related to lockdowns and infection peaks. For example, in one study of over 8,000 births in Dublin no overall change was seen in birth outcomes from January–July 2020 compared to previous years, but when data around the peak of the infection was examined a significant reduction in 'normal births' (vaginal without forceps or vacuum assistance) was found. This was mainly due to a peak in caesarean sections, with 37% of births occurring this way in data from April 2020.[28]

In terms of other labour outcomes, one study in Italy comparing interventions during labour before and during Covid-19 found an increased use of oxytocin to accelerate labour (25% versus 35%), a reduced rate of one-to-one support throughout labour, decreased mobility during labour and a lower rate of intermittent foetal monitoring (it is unclear whether less monitoring in general occurred, or whether this meant an increased rate of continuous foetal monitoring).[29] In a similar study in Scotland women were more likely to have an epidural or spinal anaesthesia during Covid then they were in comparative data from 2018 (54% versus 46%).[30] However, much research in this area is still ongoing.

In terms of the specific impacts of the changes to care and altered birth experiences on birth trauma, one study in the US compared women's rates of birth trauma before and after the pandemic, matching women by their demographic background. They measured how stressful women found childbirth using a tool called the Peritraumatic Distress Inventory, which explores feelings such as guilt, shame, helplessness, fear and horror. Women who gave birth during the pandemic exhibited a significantly higher stress response to childbirth than those who gave birth before it. This stress response was in turn related to symptoms of childbirth-related post-traumatic stress disorder, increased difficulties bonding with their baby and breastfeeding challenges.[31] Another study in Spain found significantly higher levels of a measure of stress during birth when comparing women who gave birth before or during the pandemic.[25]

Birth trauma support is vital in terms of helping women heal.[32] Women and men who are experiencing traumatic memories from a birth (including what happened to their partner) benefit from the chance to talk about their experiences and receive different therapies depending on the severity and type of their symptoms. Access to this care can make all the difference in helping traumatised parents move forward, and is valued by those who can participate. However, on top of the traumatic births they experienced, many parents then found that it was difficult to get any sort of follow-up appointment after birth to raise such issues. In one study a mother talked about being offered an opportunity for face-to-face support, but she was too anxious about contracting Covid to attend.[33]

The impact of virtual and reduced care

As we have seen, antenatal care is vitally important in helping reduce the risk of complications, improving birth outcomes and supporting maternal health and wellbeing.[1] Face-to-face care is an important part of antenatal service delivery for numerous reasons, including developing a relationship between midwife and mother, picking up on symptoms and worries, and adapting messages to the needs of families.[34] Women value appointments where they receive both physical checks and emotional support and have the time to ask questions and receive reassurance.[35]

One consequence of the pandemic was that many antenatal appointments suddenly changed – almost overnight – to be delivered over the phone or by video call. Where physical checks were necessary women often perceived these as rushed and impersonal. Some women described having to do 90% of their appointment on the phone sat outside in their car, followed by rushing into a clinic for a growth or blood pressure check.[36]

Of course it is understandable, given the circumstances of the pandemic, that it might be necessary to reduce some face-to-face appointments, but the knock-on effect also has to be recognised. The set-up described above also places some women at risk. What do you do if you don't have a car? Stand in the street while heavily pregnant and discuss your personal health on the phone while strangers walk by?

Understandably these arrangements led to women feeling that their care was impersonal, with two-thirds feeling it negatively impacted their relationship with their health professional.[36] Many did not like having appointments over the phone in particular, not just because it was less personal, but because they were worried that warning symptoms might be missed. Women found it difficult to convey physical issues over a phone call or screen. These fears were naturally stronger in those who had experienced a previous stillbirth, miscarriage or other complication. Others found the face-to-face parts of their appointments rushed, with midwives wanting them in and out as soon as possible.[33] There was little chance for reassurance or to ask questions – it was all about the physical health checks.

We also have to consider the practical implications of these changes to appointments for those in more vulnerable positions. Some women in the research noted how phone appointments were particularly challenging due to hearing impairments.[36] Others described how they now had to have phone appointments at home rather than in the privacy of the clinic. They did not necessarily want to bring up topics in front of their partner, particularly in cases of domestic abuse.

Other women had appointments reduced or cancelled altogether, which raised anxieties around complications or led to women simply feeling that they did not have enough information. In the *Babies in Lockdown* report, accessing sufficient information during pregnancy was a common issue, with 38% of participants worried about finding reliable information and advice.[37] In some cases, although standard care went ahead, additional appointments were cancelled. One woman in the report described how her appointments for specialist epilepsy care in pregnancy were cancelled indefinitely.

A lot of antenatal education classes, if offered at all, had to be delivered online. In one study in Australia, less than a third of pregnant women received any antenatal education at all, with what there was mainly delivered online.[38] In the UK many women reported that their antenatal education was initially cancelled.[39] Others reported having to seek private or freely available classes from other sources – all of which was delivered online.[40] Although women found online classes practically useful in terms of gaining some knowledge, many did not find them useful in terms of connecting with other parents, sharing experiences or making lasting friendships. The experience often left them feeling disconnected and even more isolated than if they hadn't attempted to join in the first place.[24]

Partner restrictions

Another common restriction was whether women could have their partner or another support person with them during appointments, labour or after birth. At the start of the pandemic the majority of women found that they had to attend appointments alone, including those for complications and high-risk issues. Partners were allowed to be present for the birth, but were often not allowed into the hospital until labour was established and then sent away within an hour or so after birth. This led to some women feeling pressurised to have frequent vaginal checks to see how dilated they were, not for the purpose of monitoring their baby's health and progress, but to satisfy a regulation. For other appointments such as scans, miscarriage checks, or invasive testing partners were not allowed to attend.[41]

In order to document the restrictions and how they might differ by location, a freedom of information request was sent to every maternity service in England on 24 August 2020 in relation to partner restrictions during the first peak of the pandemic.[42] Overall 81/127 trusts responded. The degree of partner exclusion across the responses was as follows:

Antenatal care
- **12-week scan: 90%**
- **20-week scan: 88%**
- **Non-routine services such as reduced foetal movements: 95%**

As the restrictions started to ease, some hospitals started to lift the ban on partners attending appointments, but this was not applied in a uniform way. By August 2020 25% of trusts were allowing partners at the 12-week scan and 38% at the second scan. However, 43% had made no move to lift restrictions, with 24% planning on reinstating them for local lockdowns.

Labour and birth
- **Allowed to be present for the birth: 100%**
- **Restrictions on when allowed to be present: 86%**

The majority of trusts allowed partners to be present for the moment of birth, but typically placed restrictions on when they were allowed to join. For example, many could not attend for induction, during the early stages of labour or for more than a couple of hours after birth. This included for home births. Overall, 20% of trusts stopped home birth, but for trusts where home births were allowed to go ahead, 48% restricted partner attendance. In their own homes!

Postnatal care
- **Restricted attendance at postnatal services: 99%**
- **Partners not allowed to attend at all: 49%**

Given the uncertainty and chaos at the start of the pandemic, some of these changes were initially understandable. We were not sure about the risks to pregnant women and babies, how severe the virus might be, or how overloaded the healthcare system would be. But as we gradually learned more, in many areas changes didn't seem to relax or alter in line with the evidence or in comparison to other services or activities in the UK which involved social contact. Indeed, the #butnotmaternity campaign was started to highlight some of the absurdities where rules had been relaxed but partner restrictions stayed. For example, in summer 2020 in England, you could meet friends at the pub, go for a meal as a group of six and merrily spend your day shopping... but not have your partner with you if you were being induced, receiving a scan for a potential miscarriage or hospitalised with an ectopic pregnancy.[41] The rules sometimes appeared to be nonsensical and depend on who was providing the service. In one study in the UK a participant described how her partner was not allowed into her NHS 20-week scan, but a private clinic in the same town let him be present.[43]

The #butnotmaternity campaign sent a letter to the Chief Executive of the NHS asking for a sensible relaxation of rules around birth partners in line with other guidelines. It shared the results of a survey by Pregnant Then Screwed of over 15,000 pregnant women and new mothers about their experiences of partner restrictions during antenatal and postnatal care. Overall:

- **90% felt that the restrictions had a negative impact on their mental health**
- **97% stated that the restrictions increased their anxiety around childbirth**
- **17.4% felt forced into vaginal examinations, with 82% feeling it was a requirement to allow their partner access to the ward**

The letter was signed by many birth organisations, academics and health professionals and urged policymakers to make use of lateral flow tests and allow partners in to give support at an earlier stage. Although changes have since been made, many took some time and even now some hospitals still have regulations about who is allowed in the birthing room and when.[41] Indeed, a quick check of Twitter for #butnotmaternity when editing this book showed me straight away that many hospitals are *still* placing limits on who can 'visit' to support someone through appointments, birth and postnatal care.

We know that support from a partner or other companion is important to women during pregnancy and birth. Good support is associated with reduced anxiety and depression during pregnancy and the postnatal period.[44] During labour partners provide information, emotional support, facilitate communication between mothers and health professionals and provide non-pharmacological pain relief such as supportive touch.[6] Support from a trusted partner is associated with increased birth satisfaction, greater confidence and fewer interventions and complications during birth. Finally, women with good support use less pharmacological pain relief and are more likely to have a baby with a higher APGAR score at birth.[45] Good partner support is basically pretty amazing.

The effects of the restrictions on partner support were multifaceted. First of all they had a major detrimental impact on women's experience of birth. In an Italian study, women were asked which aspect of their birth experience most affected their satisfaction with birth, such as care given, how they gave birth and any pain relief given. One-third of women stated that the most negative influence had been the restrictions on their partner staying.[29] Many women worried that because their partner could not attend antenatal appointments they were missing out on the opportunity to see that the pregnancy was 'real' and to bond and connect with their baby.[33]

In particular the restrictions caused loneliness and isolation in women labouring alone. In one study in Ireland, when women were asked to recount their experiences of early labour, they talked about how entering the maternity hospital on their own and having to navigate their way to the ward while contracting left them feeling anxious and tearful.[22] Although many praised the support that midwives gave them, women also wanted the support of their partner, which they saw as a different type of support that no midwife could give. They talked about simply wanting their partner to hold their hand, reassure them and just be there for them.

Others worried about their partner missing the birth due to rules around how established labour had to be in order for them to be let in. Many hospitals adopted the rule that women could not have a birth partner with them until they were in established active labour – sometimes deemed as much as 7cm dilated. Not only did women have to labour alone, but they also had to deal with feelings of anxiety and guilt about their partner missing out on seeing their baby born.[43]

The adaptations that couples made to work around and within these rules were simultaneously heart-warming and heart-breaking. As partners were not allowed in the hospital, many spent hours waiting in the car.[22] Women described spending considerable amounts of their labour walking around hospital car parks simply to be with their partner. Some felt this was almost a positive experience – the car parks were quiet and it was a lovely, sunny day. I would imagine you would feel quite differently in the cold or the rain or if you needed pain relief.

Other stories regularly popped up in the media of women actually giving birth in the hospital car park or on the way in because they'd left it as late as possible to travel as they didn't want to risk their partner not being admitted. As we saw in the previous chapter, it's likely that at a population level this avoidance of care due to anxiety about being separated from their partner contributed in part to the increase in stillbirths that we've seen. The blame for this fully lies with the mishandling of maternity restrictions and not the women so traumatised by the system and the media that they felt staying away from care was the best option.

Partners not being present during appointments was particularly distressing for women who had a history of miscarriage or complications, or for those who went on to receive bad news. In a study in the UK one woman talked about the trauma of not only receiving the news of complications alone, but then having to relay it to her partner over the phone.[43] Women experiencing complications often had to have frequent appointments, hanging around the hospital for longer periods of time, all while feeling anxious and alone.[20] Others did not want to contact their midwife when they were experiencing possible complications such as reduced foetal movement as they knew that if they needed to go into hospital they would have to go in alone without their partner.[36]

As a consequence of restrictions on partners (and indeed other aspects of care), midwives were also placed under additional pressure. Many felt that they needed to offer the emotional support that a partner would usually have given, feeling guilty about having to leave the room and woman alone, or not being able to offer as much physical reassurance as they would have liked to.[25] Others felt responsible, or received criticism from families about the rules, even though they were not the ones who made them. It was the midwives who had to tell families that they were working with that they could not receive face-to-face support or have partners present in the early stages of labour. It was the midwives who had to step in and not only increase emotional care for women labouring alone, but also support women through the negative emotions they were experiencing due to the guidelines.[46] The authors of the study that revealed these findings describe this effect on midwives as an 'occupational moral injury'.

Understandably, women often felt that the restrictions put in place were arbitrary and too rigid.[19] One good example was the rule that partners could not be present until the mother was 4cm dilated. Why 4cm? You could potentially argue that the longer a partner was in the birth room, the more chance of them spreading the virus (if they had it). But if the period of labour from 4cm onwards could last anywhere between seemingly minutes and many hours, how is that explained? And what about women who have a very slow (but intense) early stage of labour, followed by a much quicker active stage? Women with speedy labours ended up with their partners missing the birth, while other women had their partners present for hours.

Of course, partner restrictions did not only affect the partner giving birth. We have evidence that partner support during labour is not just a positive thing for the woman giving birth and ultimately her baby, but for her partner in adapting to parenthood too. Partners who are present and involved in antenatal care and during birth feel more confident and engaged with their babies. Experiencing birth together can strengthen relationships during the transition to parenthood.[47] Skin-to-skin contact after birth can enhance fathers' attachment and bonding, decrease cortisol and increase oxytocin levels.[48] Fathers often see the moment of birth as the beginning of becoming a father, connecting with their baby.[49]

One qualitative study explored the experiences of birth partners (partners and support people) of women who had given birth during the pandemic.[50] Approximately one-third were female and two-thirds male and not all were intimate partners – around 70% were the mother's partner and 30% a friend or other birth companion. Partners and support people were naturally upset at their exclusion from appointments, although many found that healthcare professionals tried to include them where possible via phone or video call. One father talked about the obstetrician taking a video of the scan that could be shared. However, partners often felt excluded, with no one asking how they were feeling about the pregnancy, birth or all the changes occurring. This was exacerbated by antenatal education often being cancelled. Even when partners could potentially attend, many had to stay home because schools or other childcare settings were closed and no one else was allowed to provide childcare for their older children.

Both partners and support people were distressed at not being able to fully support the mother giving birth. They felt that they missed out on information and guidance given in the appointments and then were not able to be present all the way through labour to support the mother. Partners felt left out that they were not involved in decisions and care, and as though it was not their baby or their responsibility. This left many feeling anxious, which was exacerbated by the unfamiliar environment. Many partners described being separated from their partner and baby soon after birth as traumatic. Partners wanted to be able to stay and care for them both, particularly in terms of supporting the mother emotionally. Many had to leave the mother distressed and go home alone. All of this affected how some partners felt during the postnatal period – detached and isolated and that they had not really contributed to the experience.

Doula restrictions

Doulas are trained professionals who provide support to women and families through pregnancy, birth and the postnatal period. They are not medical professionals and do not offer medical advice; rather they focus on emotional and practical support, helping families make informed decisions that are right for them. Some families may work with a doula predominantly during birth, whereas others may seek more intensive support through pregnancy and into the postpartum period. The majority of research that has explored the impact of doulas focuses on birth outcomes.

The support of a doula during childbirth consistently shows an impact on birth outcomes and experiences. Even in randomised controlled trials where women are allocated a doula (or not) when they give birth, positive effects on reduced caesarean section rate, duration of labour and perceived pain are seen. The use of a randomised controlled trial reduces the likelihood that these impacts are to do with things other than doula support, such as that women with more knowledge or awareness around birth, or more money to hire a doula, are simply having better birth outcomes.[51]

Why? Well we know that continuous support during labour is associated with improved birth outcomes including fewer complications and interventions and increased birth satisfaction.[52] In busy hospital wards in particular, doulas provide one-to-one emotional support during labour, also offering a familiar face and continued relationship through the perinatal period. Doula support is associated with increased confidence and feelings of control during birth, which we know are also linked to improved birth outcomes.[53] Most importantly, women who have the support of a doula are more likely to be satisfied with their birth experience than those who do not – a key feature in reducing birth trauma and postnatal depression.[54] Doula support can be particularly important when a woman has little family support, strained relationships or feels her partner will not be able to offer her the support she needs. Doulas provide support not just to the birthing mother, but can also be valuable in helping to support partners through the process.[55]

However, alongside restrictions on partner support during labour, restrictions were also put in place around whether doulas could support mothers in the hospital. They were often subject to the same restrictions as partners (e.g. not being allowed in the hospital until active labour), and mothers were often told that they had to choose between having a birth partner present and a doula. This not only deprived the mother of doula support during birth (and all the benefits just discussed), but also placed mothers in the stressful position of having to choose between a partner and a doula.

These restrictions were widespread. A survey of over 500 doulas from 23 countries conducted in March–April 2020 documented the impact of lockdown restrictions on where and how doulas were able to practise.[56] Many doulas reported that they were simply unable to attend births. Typically this was because hospitals allowed a maximum of one birth partner and placed strict limitations on postpartum visiting. Some doulas even reported that they faced similar restrictions at home births. Others found that their country/area did not class them as essential workers and that they were subject to travel restrictions or not able to enter people's homes. Some moved their doula care online, offering video calls and support, but found it much more challenging to connect with mothers, or to fully immerse themselves in support as they too had young children or working partners at home.

Doulas repeatedly tried to ask for further access to support mothers. In one study a doula talked about writing letters to the hospital and the Minister of Health explaining the benefits of her support, but with no result. Others felt frustrated that they were not able to carry out their full role, and that the hospital was dismissing the skill and care they could offer. Many felt undervalued and that they could have been of significant benefit to a system that was struggling under the pressures of the pandemic.[50]

Research from the US found that doulas worked to try and inform women about hospital policies they might encounter (such as birth positions a certain hospital might try and promote), the techniques for reducing stress during labour and visualisations around safety and a smooth delivery. Doulas were trying to protect the women they were supporting as much as possible, while themselves dealing with uncertainty and the impact of restrictions on their role. Many found it extremely frustrating that they couldn't offer the support they wanted to during birth.[57]

When doulas were allowed in to support a mother but the partner was then excluded, even if that was what the parents had chosen together, some doulas were left with feelings of guilt about the partner missing out. Sometimes they felt uneasy and uncomfortable, especially if it was a first birth and they felt that the mother and partner potentially did not realise what they were missing out on. This was exacerbated by some midwives expressing surprise that the doula was there instead of the partner. However, some doulas reassured themselves that they had been actively chosen by the mother, usually because of previous trauma or a known need for additional support. The doula knew that they were the person best placed in that scenario to be able to support the mother.[50]

At the time of writing many doulas are still not allowed in the birth room with both parents. They could go clubbing with the expectant parents, but not with them into the hospital!

Restricting birth options

Aside from restrictions on support during birth, other birthing options were restricted in a number of ways. Two prime examples were restrictions by some trusts on requests for maternal caesarean by choice, and the use of water for pain relief. These restrictions had the potential to affect women in two main ways: firstly, by removing the benefits that they had decided that those birth options would offer them, and secondly, by removing their right to make informed decisions about their care.

Some trusts restricted maternal caesarean by choice, arguing that it could potentially mean a longer hospital stay, an increased need for post-birth care and a greater use of healthcare resources. However, that rationale appears to assume that if a woman is not granted an elective section she will automatically give birth vaginally without complications. This has been challenged.[58] Women do not tend to make a request for a caesarean section lightly. Physical health complications or significant psychological distress are typically at the heart of these requests. Fears around the impact of labour and vaginal birth on complications such as symphysis pubis dysfunction, pelvic floor issues or pre-existing digestive disorders are common. Many requests are made due to previous psychological birth trauma. These aspects are significant in themselves, but the added removal of informed decision-making, choice and autonomy can exacerbate anxieties, which in turn increase the risk of complications during childbirth. To remove an option from a woman who is significantly distressed by the thought of labour and vaginal delivery removes dignity and is inhumane.

NICE guidelines support the use of water during birth, but state that the evidence is insufficient to actively encourage it. This appears to be because studies that focus on the 'hard' outcomes of birth, such as maternal or infant morbidity or mortality, show no difference between water births and those out of water.[59]

However, reviews that consider woman-centred factors reveal that water birth can help reduce some other labour complications, such as perineal trauma and post-partum haemorrhage.[60] Meanwhile, women who have had a water birth perceive the experience as empowering, as increasing their control and autonomy, and helpful in supporting them to cope with labour pain. These seem like pretty significant outcomes if we actually care about the experiences of women during and after birth, rather than just the physiological severe outcomes.[61]

Water is an important means of pain relief and relaxation for women who want it during labour. Several studies from around the world, including the UK, Australia and Holland, reported restrictions being placed on water births.[60,62,63] In a UK study exploring women's experiences of birth, 10% were told they could not have a water birth due to Covid restrictions (although not all women would have requested one).[64] In another study in Australia a midwife described how there was pressure put on them at one point to try to stop women having a water birth in their own homes.[65] The reasons for this were unclear. Some guidelines, including those from the Royal College of Obstetricians and Gynaecologists, specifically stated that water birth should not be used when a woman was positive for Covid-19, due to evidence of the virus in faeces and midwives not being able to wear full PPE. However, there was no reason why women who had not tested positive should not have one.[66]

Restrictions on water birth had a significant negative impact on the anxiety and wellbeing levels of pregnant women who were hoping to use water to cope with their labour. In one study a woman talked about how not being able to have a water birth 'severely impacted' her pregnancy, leaving her feeling anxious and unsupported.[67] I would imagine this distress was multifaceted. Yes her pain relief option had been taken away, but so had her feelings of control and security, which we could argue may well have more influence on her birth experience.

The impact of home birth restrictions

Home births were suspended in over a third of trusts in England. Reasons given for suspension included reduced staffing, a need to redirect any resources towards Covid-19 and ambulance shortages.[68] However, in a review paper entitled '*Home birthing in the United Kingdom during Covid-19*' the authors examine how these decisions not only impacted on choice and wellbeing, but may also have inadvertently led to women deciding to birth outside of the system without medical care. Legally, the situation regarding offering home births or not is complex. There is no law to say you can automatically have one. But likewise there is no law to say you need to go to hospital. You are allowed to refuse medical treatment. Midwives have a professional obligation to attend a birth at home that they have become aware of.[58]

The reasons for choosing a home birth are varied and include previous negative hospital experiences, birth trauma, wanting to reduce the likelihood of unnecessary interventions and/or increase the likelihood of having a straightforward delivery, and a simple desire to want to give birth in a place that feels familiar and comfortable. The birth trauma aspect is particularly important.

Many second time or more mothers turn to home birth after feeling so traumatised by a negative hospital experience that they cannot bear to re-enter the hospital to give birth.[69]

Research has shown that for low-risk women planned home birth carries a lower risk of interventions and complications such as caesarean section, foetal dystocia, perineal trauma and post-partum haemorrhage. Where studies are high quality and control for other factors, no difference occurs in infant mortality between home and hospital.[70] Women who give birth at home report perceived better quality care and more satisfaction with their birth experience.[71] Home birth may also be more cost effective than hospital birth – one economic analysis in the US found that having an additional 10% of deliveries take place in private homes or freestanding birth centres could safely save almost $11 billion per year.[72]

So home birth is a logical choice for low-risk women who feel comfortable birthing at home. Throw in a pandemic, high levels of fear about the safety of hospitals and restrictions around partners entering the hospital... and it is unsurprising that some women wanted a home birth more than ever. Indeed, in one study with privately practising midwives in Australia, 93% reported an increase in the number of enquiries relating to home birth. Some midwives reported an increase of over 20 extra calls per month, with some coming as late as 39 weeks of pregnancy. Given that home birth rates in Australia are typically low, at around 0.3%, this is significant – one midwife compared the volume of calls she had received in the last week to the number she typically received in six months. Reasons for women wanting a home birth included concerns about changes to care during labour due to Covid-19 protocols, increased Covid-19 exposure, and limited birth partner support.[73]

Where home births remained available, rates rapidly increased. One study in Ontario, Canada, saw a rise from around 13% of births occurring at home to 20% in May 2020.[74] In Australia around 30% of women reported changing their preferred birth place plans, with the majority wanting to move from a hospital to a home birth.[75] Reports from one publicly funded home birth programme in Victoria, Australia, showed that home births tripled in March–May 2020 compared to previous years.[76] Finally, another study in the US found that women were changing to home births, with 5.4% of women in their study wanting a home birth compared to a national average of 1.6% before the pandemic. The reasons for now wanting a home birth included restrictions on birth partners, restrictions on postnatal visitors and fear about the virus. Others found their planned childcare for older children during the birth was affected by lockdown restrictions, meaning that their partner would have to stay at home rather than being with them at the hospital.[77]

Notably, the option to have a home birth may have protected women's mental health. In one US-based study that compared pregnant women's anxieties before and during the pandemic, those planning a home birth had the smallest increase in anxiety scores during the pandemic. The authors attribute this to fewer concerns about infection, alongside the reassurance of being able to take control of the situation. Conversely, those who felt unsure about where they would now give birth showed some of the highest increases in anxiety. In this study rates of women planning a hospital birth dropped from 96% pre-pandemic to 87% during it.[78]

Many health decisions can have unintended consequences, and one consequence of placing restrictions on partner presence and birth options, and then shutting down home birth provision, was a rise in the number of women considering or actually giving birth outside a hospital setting without any health professional support – a practice known as free birthing. While technically legal, free birthing (when compared to home birth with a midwife) can carry an increased risk of complications during labour and birth because of the lack of monitoring and professional support.

However, many women who choose to free birth end up feeling it is the least risky situation for them due to previous traumatic birth experiences or negative experiences with antenatal care.[79]

Fears around giving birth in a hospital started to rise in relation to media messages around risk combined with changes to birth care. Articles in the press highlighted how women felt safer outside of the system.[80] For example, in a study in the UK that explored how the first lockdown affected women's experiences of antenatal care, 72 of the 1,700 women who responded said that they had seriously considered free birthing rather than giving birth in a hospital. Notably, just one participant stated that they had been planning on free birthing before the pandemic occurred – although this cannot be directly compared as it was not a 'before and after' study. Most had planned a home birth or to give birth in a midwife-led unit – these decisions were now under threat. Others had hoped to hire an independent midwife to give birth at home, but found that everyone was fully booked up because suddenly more women were in the same position.

Reasons for choosing free birth included broader reasons than Covid-19, such as previous birth trauma, fear of hospitals, worries about interventions or coercion or practical reasons such as a lack of transport or childcare. Notably these are also reasons why women typically choose a home birth – removing the home birth option appears to potentially push women into free birthing rather than agreeing to go to hospital. However a number of reasons were more specifically related to Covid-19: worries about birth partners being excluded, water births being banned or fear of contracting Covid-19.[81]

Postnatal ward restrictions

Visitors were severely restricted on most postnatal wards. Many women experienced their partner being sent home straight after birth, with some allowed to return only at designated visiting hours for a short period of time, although different hospitals appeared to implement different rules. Other visitors were not allowed. This separation and isolation is one of the most distressing findings to emerge from research into parenting and the pandemic. In the *Babies in Lockdown* report, many new mothers talked about being separated from their partner during early labour and induction and then them being sent home as soon as the baby was born.[37]

Understandably this had an impact on mothers, affected by how long they needed to stay after the birth. Some women could see a positive side to having fewer visitors on the ward (especially fewer of other people's visitors). In one study with new mothers in Ireland women did feel an additional layer of connection to other women in the postnatal ward, sharing stories and forging friendships in a way they felt they would not have if things had been different. Some also talked about breastfeeding in the early days being easier because there were fewer interruptions from visitors.[22]

However, other women really struggled with feelings of loneliness and isolation, including feeling guilty if they had to stay in hospital any longer than the minimum as their partner could not see their baby. Many sent regular videos and photos but felt a pressure to try and maintain some kind of connection between their partner and baby. Women should not be feeling this additional pressure after having a baby while they are recovering in hospital.[22]

Postnatal ward restrictions also led to women wanting to discharge themselves as soon as possible after the birth. In some research we did during the first lockdown exploring mothers' experiences of breastfeeding, we found that many missed out on breastfeeding support in those early hours or even gave their baby formula when they didn't really want to, just to get home.[82] This was also reflected in the *Babies in Lockdown* report, with mothers being sent home quickly without any sort of feeding plan. Feeding support was then given over the phone if needed.[37]

Others struggled with an absence of visitors because visitors often did small tasks such as pouring drinks or passing things to the mother if she was in a lot of pain. This meant that mothers had to rely on staff, who were already overstretched. Visitors do so much more on a ward than simply provide emotional support. While you can talk to your partner over video call, they can't pass you your baby if you're immobilised after a difficult birth.[43]

The impact of PPE, social distancing and cleaning

Given the concerns around infection during labour and birth, especially due to the necessity of close contact, personal protective equipment (PPE) was required for midwives and sometimes recommended or required for women and their partners. This was important for protecting health professionals, who may come into contact with many families, and its need for staff is clear. However, this doesn't mean that it didn't have any unintended consequences for women's experiences during labour and birth – and indeed for staff themselves.

In terms of women themselves being required to wear PPE during labour and birth, guidance appeared to differ or be interpreted differently by hospitals in the UK and other countries. In one UK study 14.5% of women reported that they were asked to wear a mask or another form of PPE themselves during labour.[43] In another study in Italy at the start of the pandemic, on entering the ward mothers were tested for Covid-19. All women were required to wear a mask during labour. If the result was not returned by the time their baby was born, they had to wear a surgical mask and gloves to breastfeed their baby. Partners were allowed to be present during labour and for two hours after birth, but had to wear a surgical mask, gloves, cap, overshoes and coat.[29]

In terms of the impact of staff needing to wear masks and additional PPE, experiences have been mixed. Some women have reported that it made them feel safer, both for themselves and because they felt reassured that those caring for them weren't being put at risk. However, others found it made them feel unsettled or that it made communicating more difficult.[43] This was echoed in an Italian study. Some women were reassured by staff wearing PPE, seeing it as a sign that their hospital was prepared, professional and taking measures to keep them safe. Others felt that PPE signified danger, and they wanted to discharge themselves from the hospital as soon as possible.[83] And finally, in one study two pregnant mothers who had a hearing impairment were worried about not being able to understand staff and communicate their needs when everyone was wearing a mask.[36]

Midwives have also spoken about how distressing caring for labouring women while wearing full PPE and trying to keep their distance has been.[84] They had to try and rely on using their eyes to convey support, rather than being able to touch, hug and comfort physically, with some describing the situation as 'dehumanised'. Others struggled with the discomfort of their PPE, particularly during warmer months, adapting their behaviour to spend more time outside of birth rooms – during induction for example – so that they could have a break. Another detail is that the time spent putting on and taking off PPE, although short, soon added up across midwives on the ward, reducing the time available for supporting women.

The effect on midwives of the pandemic and changes to maternity care

It was of course not just the impact of PPE that was distressing for midwives, and we will return to the significant challenges that the pandemic has had for them, alongside health visitors, other healthcare workers and volunteers throughout this book. These additional pressures and stresses came at a time when the profession was already under considerable strain due to staff shortages, burnout and demoralisation, creating a perfect storm of distress for many. Even before the pandemic, a survey of nearly 2,000 midwives in the UK reported that 83% of those who responded were experiencing moderate symptoms of personal burnout and 67% work-related burnout. Over a third were experiencing symptoms of moderate or more severe stress, or clinically significant symptoms of anxiety or depression.[85] As I write, reports have revealed that England is experiencing a critical shortage of midwives, with almost 2,500 fewer midwives in post than are needed.[86] The pandemic may have exacerbated this, but staffing was already at critical levels before we had even heard of Covid-19.

How did the pandemic and restrictions affect those caring for families? In multiple ways, as a critical report published by the Royal College of Midwives highlighted early in the pandemic.[87] Firstly midwives, like many health and social care professionals, had to manage fears about the personal risk to them and their families of Covid-19 infection. Those at increased risk of infection due to pregnancy or coming from BAME backgrounds felt heightened fear, as did those affected by an initial lack of PPE.[88]

In terms of caregiving, many struggled with some of the institutional changes proposed, feeling powerless to make a stand or care for women in the way that they wanted to. They could see harm occurring to those they were caring for (and they knew how care now differed compared to pre-Covid-19 times, even if parents were unaware). As we have seen, it was the health professionals who had to follow through with these changes and be the 'messenger' to distressed families.

Instructions to reduce physical contact were particularly challenging. For example, in one global study of 127 midwives, obstetricians, and other healthcare workers from 71 different countries, many talked about the challenges and depersonalisation of trying to keep their distance from women.[89] When physical checks were needed, midwives were often instructed to do them as quickly as possible, knowing how impersonal this would feel for the women. Midwives missed being able to engage sensitively with mothers, both during intimate examinations and more broadly in terms of providing reassurance. They could not reach out and hug or soothe a woman in the same way as they were used to. In some countries physical examinations such as cervical dilation or foetal heartbeat monitoring were carried out at much longer intervals than is recommended, potentially placing mothers and babies at risk.

In the same study participants also talked about how other measures kept them physically distant from women, which also created further emotional distance. For example, some reported policies of sending women home if they were not in established labour, whereas they would usually have kept them on the ward for support if they needed it. In addition, the increased cleaning requirements meant that some hospitals limited how much women could move about during labour. Some stated that they must stay on the bed, while others stated that they must not leave the room or ward. This prevented pain-relief options such as having a bath during labour, or walking around to ease pain and encourage the progression of labour. Others reported that space on wards designed to support labouring women was repurposed for Covid-19 related support, or for storage of furniture or equipment not currently in use as other areas of the hospital were dedicated to Covid-19 support.

Other aspects, such as the shortage of staff, meant that healthcare professionals had to focus on the most pressing issues, which often meant reduced time spent with mothers simply supporting them. This was particularly challenging when caring for a woman in labour who was positive for Covid-19, as staff could not move around and support multiple women as needed – they had to solely care for the infected mother. This led to cases of midwives caring for women on their own at crucial points where two midwives would usually be present.

The impact of these changes in regulations was draining for staff. Some felt that all the requirements resulted in them struggling to be supportive and woman-centred in the care that they gave as they felt so fraught and uncomfortable. Many struggled with changing guidelines and not being sure what policy was currently in place or the justification behind it, not helped by communication feeling more challenging due to the wearing of PPE and social distancing. This was particularly challenging when families asked staff to explain the new regulations. This significant additional 'emotional load' on caregivers must not be underestimated.

Indeed, in other studies from around the world, the psychological impact on midwives of simply trying to do their job and care for women and families is emerging. One study of 758 nurses and midwives in Turkey showed that many were experiencing mental health difficulties related to the pandemic. Two-thirds were feeling anxious and uncertain, with almost half feeling that they needed psychological support. Twelve per cent were so distressed by the situation that they wanted to leave.[90] This is echoed in studies of other health professionals which we will return to later.

Looking at more clinical measures of mental health, in one Australian study almost a third of midwives reported symptoms of anxiety.[91] In another Turkish study a third of nurses and midwives had clinical symptoms of depression, with the risk of depression almost double in midwives compared to nurses. This suggests that it is not simply the impact of increased workload and anxiety of working in healthcare during the pandemic that has affected midwives, but also having to so drastically adapt the style of care given.[92]

Assessing the impact of these changes

Changes to care (advised or otherwise) were ultimately put in place with the intention of reducing transmission of the virus, to protect both healthcare professionals and parents. Combined with the impact on staffing that affected the provision of some services, it is clear that many families in maternity services were significantly affected by the regulations. Sadly, the impact of some of these changes and their knock-on effects, alongside the increased maternal anxiety discussed in the previous chapter, has now been implicated in some maternal and infant deaths during the pandemic.

The Healthcare Safety Investigation Branch (HSIB) conducts investigations into how healthcare practices may have harmed NHS patients, including those in maternity services. It has produced a number of reports examining morbidity and mortality during the pandemic that was not directly related to Covid-19 infection. Two reports in particular are relevant here: one examining the context surrounding maternal deaths and one examining the circumstances surrounding stillbirths. Both reports focus on how changes to care had unintended negative consequences for the care mothers sought and were given.

The first report examines the context surrounding maternal death investigations during the first wave of the Covid-19 pandemic and attributes seven changes to maternal deaths during this period.[93] These were:

1. Unprecedented demand for telephone health advice causing delays in accessing healthcare: women often struggled to get through to healthcare professionals when they had concerns or urgent issues.

2. Public messaging and 'safety netting' advice causing delays in seeking healthcare: women delayed or avoided attending hospital due to fear of catching the virus and/or being separated from their partner.

3. Guidance changing rapidly: hospitals and staff were often unclear as to the most up-to-date guidance.

4. Use of early warning scores did not always detect deterioration: essentially, clinical observations and tests used to check health did not work, most likely due to an increase in virtual appointments.

5. **Personal protective equipment requirements changing due to Covid-19: PPE changes took up time, reducing time spent with women, increased communication difficulties and errors, and subsequently heightened stress levels.**
6. **Staff described feelings of stress and distress which can affect performance: communication difficulties, redeployment and reduced staffing increased staff stress and therefore impacted upon care.**
7. **Difficulties in making a diagnosis and choosing treatment strategies: little was known about the development and progression of Covid-19 in pregnant women. This was enhanced by fears around infection, a lack of face-to-face contact and delays in testing.**

The second report examines the context surrounding stillbirths referred to HSIB in April–June 2020, specifically for those where a baby was alive at the start of labour but was born with no signs of life.[94] HSIB noticed an almost twofold increase in this type of referral compared to the same period in 2019, and conducted an examination into whether Covid-19 related care factors were responsible. Notably Covid-19 infections were not present in any of these cases, suggesting direct issues with care rather than complications of infection. The report identified six key concerns:

1. **Challenges in interpreting and ensuring consistent implementation of rapidly changing national guidance in relation to Covid-19.**
2. **Issues with risk management where trusts over emphasised the risks of Covid-19 compared to known existing risks around pregnancy and care, i.e. by implementing remote consultations that increased the risk of warning signs being missed.**
3. **Use of telephone triage increased communication difficulties and challenges in accessing records. Partners were excluded**

from appointments.
4.   Issues with interpretation services not being present, exacerbated by women having to attend appointments alone.
5.   Increased work demands on healthcare professionals, alongside reduced capacity to respond, decreased care given.
6.   Significant variability in neonatal resuscitation between hospital trusts. With relation to Covid-19 this was affected by changes to clinical environment and staffing.

Ultimately it is now clear that overly restrictive regulations around antenatal and birth care, alongside heightened anxiety, impacted on parental emotional wellbeing and access to and experience of care. In some cases this had a catastrophic effect on maternal and infant mortality. We must ensure that all valued services are reinstated and support both new parents and those caring for them to recover and heal from traumatic experiences during this time.

3

GIVING BIRTH WHILE POSITIVE FOR COVID-19

GIVING BIRTH WHILE
POSITIVE FOR COVID-19

It is undeniable that experiences of labour and birth were changed for many families, but a particular impact was seen on women who tested positive for Covid-19 either before birth or on entry to the hospital. We've already looked at the impact of Covid-19 infection on physical birth outcomes in Chapter 1, but what did it mean in terms of the ways women were cared for and experienced labour and birth?

At the start of the pandemic recommendations were made as to how pregnant and new mothers with Covid-19 should be cared for. The World Health Organization explicitly stated in April 2020 that:

- **Skin-to-skin should still occur**
- **Breastfeeding should still occur**
- **Mother and baby should not be separated**
- **Mothers should practise hand washing and wear a mask**

This guidance was put in place based on the balance of evidence of risk of Covid-19 to infants versus the risk of separation from their mother and not being breastfed. Skin-to-skin contact offers numerous benefits for infants, including helping to regulate their temperature, breathing and heart rate. It is also associated with a longer duration of breastfeeding.[2] Likewise, keeping mother and baby together after birth supports positive attachment between mother and baby and is also associated with a longer duration of breastfeeding.[3]

In terms of infant feeding, as considered in greater detail in Chapter 6, breastfeeding not only protects the health of mother and baby,[4] but in a mother infected with Covid-19 provides her infant with antibodies and therefore protection against the virus via breast milk. Although a handful of studies have shown the presence of the Covid virus in breastmilk, these instances tend to be rare and often potentially due to the handling of samples by an infected mother (i.e. the virus was transferred to the milk from her, not her milk). Importantly, this detection has not been shown to actually represent a virus that is capable of replicating and infecting other cells.[5] Breastfeeding was specifically supported because while expressed breastmilk can offer the infant protection, it can be an overwhelming and exhausting process for new mothers, especially if they are themselves unwell. Breastfeeding an infant who is able to breastfeed directly is often more straightforward.[6]

Conversely, failing to follow WHO guidance by separating mother and baby and preventing skin-to-skin or breastfeeding puts infants at risk – most likely greater risk than their risk of contracting and being unwell from Covid-19, especially if mothers followed hygiene principles. It deprives infants of the security of their mother and the opportunity for responsive care – something that we know is associated with positive emotional, social and physical development. Separating mother and baby and creating breastfeeding challenges also places mothers at increased risk of postnatal depression and breastfeeding grief, at a time when they are most likely vulnerable from their experiences of Covid-19 infection and giving birth without partner support.[7]

Nonetheless, health organisations appeared to create their own versions of this clear guidance from the WHO. In a paper examining how guidance documents on the care of infants whose mothers were suspected or confirmed as having Covid-19 from 33 different countries compared to the WHO recommendations, significant disparities were found.[8] Overall, no document fully followed all WHO guidance. The most common changes were to keep babies distanced from their mothers and encourage the expressing of breastmilk rather than direct breastfeeding. Specifically, across the policies for confirmed Covid-19 infection in terms of skin-to-skin contact, 27% recommended it, 45% did not recommend it, and 27% had no information. For direct breastfeeding 48% recommended it, 48% did not recommend it and 3% had no information. Policies for what to do if Covid-19 was suspected but not yet confirmed were very similar. In terms of infant proximity, 36% of policies recommended unrestricted rooming-in, 18% recommended rooming-in but with the baby at least two metres away from the mother, and 27% recommended no rooming-in at all. Others had no information, with 3% specifying that rooming-in should be allowed if the mother requested it, suggesting that perhaps the default was to separate.

The American Academy of Paediatrics, for example, suggested that mother and baby should be separated and then, if the mother insisted on remaining with her baby, her baby should be placed six feet away from her or separated by a curtain.[9] Expressing breastmilk should be encouraged rather than direct feeding. However, this was thankfully later updated. Language used in hospital policies was often loaded with emotion. For example, one maternity unit policy in New Jersey stated: '*If separation of the infant was* refused *by a family, asymptomatic neonates were* allowed *to room in with their mother'*... as if mothers were being difficult in insisting on care recommended by the World Health Organization that would give their baby the best possible chance of protection![10]

That document from New Jersey is a 'good' example of how regulations were twisted to separate mother and baby. Other recommendations included things such as:

- If a mother insisted on staying with her baby there should be physical separation of six feet between mother and baby including where possible the use of barriers such as curtains
- The mother was not allowed to visit her baby if the baby was taken to the neonatal unit, even if the baby was isolated there
- If a symptomatic mother was tested for Covid but had not yet received the result she should be recommended to stay separate from her baby
- If the mother tested positive ideally the baby should 'be carried wherever possible by a healthy asymptomatic adult who was without Covid-19, did not have contact with a Covid-19 patient, and was without symptoms of Covid-19 for the previous 14 days. Ideally, that person would be aged less than 65 years and free of risk factors for severe Covid-19 disease.'

The distress that following these procedures would be likely to cause, through separation of a mother from her baby, the likely negative impact upon breastfeeding, and generally the increased fear that this type of risk messaging elicits would be significant – but most of all, *unnecessary*. On top of this, it has to be questioned whether separation of mother and baby actually significantly reduced any risk to the infant. Given the low incidence of infection (especially serious infection) in mothers who followed hygiene procedures, what is being risked and what is being prevented? Additionally, the infant may still become unwell, but from contact with health professionals caring for Covid positive mothers, or indeed an asymptomatic parent who has spent time with the mother. And finally, under many policies, mother and infant were reunited while she was still potentially infectious, but sufficient time had passed to damage breastfeeding and mother-infant connection. This presents a real risk of the mother still being infectious but no longer able to protect her infant via breastmilk.[11]

Impact on breastfeeding

Predictably, mothers who were Covid-19 positive and separated from their baby were less likely to continue breastfeeding compared to those who remained with their baby. One study found that babies separated from their mothers were more likely to have been given formula milk in hospital (82%) compared to those remaining with their mothers (28%). At the time of the study babies were 2–10 weeks old. Exclusive breastfeeding rates were higher among those who stayed with their mother (28%) compared to those separated (12%), while 8% of those who stayed together were exclusively formula feeding compared to 35% of those separated.[12] A similar pattern emerged from a study in Spain, in which almost half of infants of Covid positive mothers were separated, with many taken to neonatal care.[13]

Meanwhile, in a global study of mothers who had confirmed or suspected Covid-19 infection a clear impact on birth practices was seen. In the study researchers compared birth practices for those women who had symptoms at the time of birth versus later (and therefore did not have symptoms at birth).[14] They found that:

- **50% of those without Covid-19 did not have skin-to-skin for at least an hour after birth, compared to 61% who were Covid-19 positive**
- **14% of those without Covid-19 had their baby taken away from them directly after birth, compared to 29% who were Covid-19 positive**
- **6% of those without Covid-19 did not breastfeed directly at birth compared to 29% who were Covid-19 positive**
- **9% of those without Covid-19 did not have their baby stay within arm's reach on the postnatal ward compared to 40% who were Covid-19 positive**

Nearly one-third of mothers who had their baby taken away due to Covid-19 infection were unable to establish breastfeeding once they were returned, with mothers understandably experiencing considerable distress. Overall, babies were less likely to be exclusively breastfed by three months if they had been taken to a separate room rather than staying with their mother, if skin-to-skin did not happen, and if they were not directly breastfed. Notably no difference was found in the rate of infant Covid-19 infection dependent on whether skin-to-skin occurred, the baby stayed with their mother, or whether babies were directly breastfed or given expressed breastmilk. With hygiene precautions in place these data suggest no impact of separating mother and baby on Covid-19 infection risk. Ultimately greater harm overall was caused by separation.

This is a stark but unsurprising conclusion. We know how important breastmilk is for premature and sick babies and policies are in place to encourage and support mothers to establish their milk supply and to enable their babies to receive as much human milk as possible.[15] But establishing a good milk supply after a premature birth, which may carry an increased likelihood of complications and more than likely be very stressful, can be challenging from a physiological and psychological perspective. We know that birth interventions, including prematurity, are associated with a greater likelihood of delayed milk production. Sick and premature babies may be unable to latch directly on to the breast, meaning that milk needs to be expressed. It is far more challenging to express milk than it is for a baby to stimulate milk supply by feeding directly from the breast. Although stress doesn't impact directly upon milk production, it can interfere with 'let down' (how easily milk is released from the milk ducts in the breast).

Many of the things that help a mother establish a good milk supply after a premature or distressing birth are erased by separation. Many women find it easier to express milk when next to their baby, or while (or after) holding their baby skin-to-skin. Likewise, once a baby is stronger, holding them skin-to-skin and letting them root for a nipple, even if they can't fully latch, helps them on their journey to fully feeding. Support, reassurance and encouragement from nurses and midwives on the neonatal ward can be incredibly helpful. Keeping stress to a minimum helps. Separating a mother from her vulnerable newborn baby is the antithesis of all this.[16]

In low and middle-income countries, many of which did implement restrictions on mother and baby staying together, the impact on breastfeeding may have been life-threatening. The importance of breastfeeding becomes more critical when we are talking about babies in developing countries where access to formula milk, sanitation and clean water is more variable. We know that globally 800,000 babies die each year due to not being exclusively breastfed, the vast majority in these regions are due to preventable infection. One study used a tool that estimates the impact of infant feeding on infant and maternal outcomes in different countries known as the 'Lives Saved Tool'.[17] This estimated that in low and middle-income countries the potential number of infant deaths due to Covid-19 during 2020–21 might be in the range of 1,800–2,800 deaths globally. In contrast, if mothers in these countries with confirmed Covid-19 infection were told to stop breastfeeding, the estimated infant death toll would be in the range of 188,000–273,000.

Impact on mothers

Understandably, giving birth while positive for Covid-19 was a distressing experience for mothers, even those who were well enough to care for their babies. In one study in Italy, women who had tested positive for Covid-19 and were 'allowed' to breastfeed their baby reported high levels of anxiety due to concerns being raised around transmission. They worried about holding their babies for longer than was 'necessary' and tried to keep feeds to a minimum.[18] In a Chinese study mothers who tested positive for Covid-19 and were separated from their babies had lower mother–child attachment scores.[19] Finally, in one study over half of mothers who gave birth while Covid-19 positive showed signs of clinical trauma after birth. This was exacerbated by a lack of partner support during labour and separation from their baby after birth.[20]

Women's experiences of birth were significantly changed too. A study in the US examined the impact of giving birth while positive for Covid-19. One major difference in experience was that women were not allowed their partner with them at all during the birth or on the postnatal ward. Additionally, their baby was less likely to be able to stay with them after birth, partly because of increased admissions to neonatal care. Compared to women giving birth who were not positive, women with Covid-19 reported higher levels of pain during delivery. They were six times more likely to report high levels of stress during birth than those who were not positive.[21]

Another study in northern Italy highlighted the devastating impact of receiving a positive test, particularly at the start of the pandemic when anxiety was particularly high.[18] A central feeling was a sense of chaos and uncertainty. Women found that their healthcare professionals were unsure what to do or about what would happen, which felt extremely unsettling. No one could be sure about the safety of the baby or what would happen after the baby was born. This was exacerbated by misinformation and horror stories flying around in the media, deliberately trying to stir up fear.

One woman talked about her experience of attending an antenatal appointment at the hospital but testing positive and not being allowed back home. Instead, she was immediately transported to an unfamiliar 'referral centre' alone, via an ambulance. No details were given about how long she would be there, and women were unable to take any of their belongings with them. Many of these centres were far from women's homes. Not even partners (who they had been living with until that point) could visit.

Others ended up staying in hospital for significant durations, with their partners unable to be present with them during labour. Sometimes women received the news that they were positive during early labour, and immediately they feared for the safety of their baby, being separated from them after birth and whether they would be able to breastfeed. Their partners, who were waiting to come and join them, were suddenly no longer allowed in, with women then worrying about their partner missing out and feeling guilty. Others feared that they would pass the infection to midwives, and felt guilty about needing support. Some felt guilty about their baby's birth experience, in that they couldn't kiss or cuddle them in the way they hoped.

Many described the care they received while Covid positive as professional and caring, but also sometimes staff responded in very clinical or brusque ways. One woman described how staff would keep telling her to stay away from them, and would tell her where to stand. She was woken in the morning at 6am by someone yelling 'masks' at her from the doorway, describing it as if she was in an army barracks. Others knew that staff were deliberately reducing the time they spent with them, in part because they had to dress in full PPE, which made them feel like a burden.

When women's babies were born their trauma often continued. If a baby tested positive they were usually taken away to neonatal intensive care and mothers were not allowed to visit them. This was clearly traumatic for the mother of the baby, but also for other mothers on the postnatal ward, who described watching someone come in and suddenly remove a baby from their mother. Women whose babies were taken to neonatal care talked about the immense guilt that they felt for not being able to be there with their baby, even though they were not allowed entry. They talked about feeling empty and like 'not a good enough mother' or like they had abandoned their baby despite it being out of their control. Others had to wear gloves to handle their baby, and were not allowed to kiss them. Some had to remain on the postnatal ward, without their baby, alongside women who had their baby next to them.

Understandably, many women in the study retained long-lasting negative memories about their experience of giving birth. One mother described how she could not look at photos taken at the hospital without crying. Others talked about their experience leaving 'scars'. Seeing or being reminded of the hospital also brought back awful memories. One mother even talked about having a second child in the future in order to experience the positives that she could not have with her baby during the pandemic. Many women in the study cried and showed visible signs of distress during their interviews, noting that they had never explained fully how they felt before because it was too emotionally distressing or they did not want to burden others.

The impact of caring for women diagnosed as Covid-19 positive should also not be underestimated.[22] In a UK study with midwives feelings of shock and concern for themselves if a woman tested positive, alongside anxiety and empathy for the woman they were caring for, were common. Many hospitals routinely tested women on entry, with tests taking some time to come back at the start of the pandemic. This meant that sometimes well and asymptomatic women tested positive – which came as a complete shock to everyone. Often this was suddenly announced and care staff had to back away from the woman, whose birth plans were then rapidly altered. Many described these scenes as chaotic and traumatic.

Impact on partners

The impact on fathers and partners of their partner giving birth while Covid positive should also not be underestimated. We have so much evidence about the importance of partner support for the birthing mother, but partners themselves are also affected by pregnancy and birth experiences. Not only is it part of their transition to becoming a parent (or a parent again), but they are also affected by seeing their partner suffering or knowing she is unsupported. As noted previously, research with fathers finds that in traumatic situations around pregnancy and birth, many feel that they have to be the strong one, who their partner can rely on.

As part of the study that explored women's experiences of giving birth while positive for Covid-19, the research team interviewed fourteen partners (who were all male/fathers).[18] No data was available on whether partners themselves had tested positive, as testing was only available for pregnant women at the time, but all had to isolate due to their partner being positive. Overall, fathers had concerns about the virus itself, the impact on their partner and baby, and their own experience of the birth. As with mothers, many of the fathers, prior to their partner's infection, were anxious about contracting Covid-19 in case it meant that they missed the birth. Many took additional measures such as wearing masks and gloves (before these were made mandatory) and showering and washing all clothes on return from work. This included anxiety about themselves missing the experience, but also predominantly not being able to be there for their partner.

Fathers found the physical (and often abrupt) separation from their partner traumatic. Some tried to catch a glimpse of their partner through the maternity ward windows, or hung around in the car park hoping they might spot her. Many did not and were left feeling empty and alone. The feeling of not being able to be there for their partner and 'protect' her and their baby was strong. Men felt a strong sense of duty and responsibility and subsequent guilt at letting their partner down, despite this being outside of their control.

Not being able to be present at the birth was traumatic for fathers, with many using words such as 'nightmare' and 'disastrous' to describe their experience. They felt as if their transition to parenthood had been delayed, and they had been denied the experience of being present for the birth. One described trying to contact the maternity ward and when he got through being told that his son had already been born. Fathers found the separation from their partner during labour distressing, not knowing what was going on. Many sat waiting in the car for hours, trying to find out information. One tried to support his partner through video call during the birth but could only hear her distress while he stared at the ceiling.

When fathers finally could 'meet' their baby, this often had to be done via video call, which some were apprehensive about doing, wanting their first time to be in person. One father even described how a midwife brought the baby to the wall on the ground floor so he could hear her cry. Sometimes, if mothers were still within the infection period even when she could go home, the reunion was marred by having to socially distance and wear masks until it passed.

Overall, overly cautious misinterpretation of guidelines led (and continues in some cases to lead) to separation of mothers and babies despite clinical evidence and policy that they should have remained together. We must always ensure that mothers and babies are viewed and treated as a dyad rather than separate entities. Although risk from Covid-19 infection must be managed, we must always ensure that harms from unnecessary separation are recognised and a balance of care given.

EXPERIENCING PREGNANCY COMPLICATIONS DURING THE PANDEMIC

EXPERIENCING PREGNANCY
COMPLICATIONS DURING
THE PANDEMIC

We looked at the impact of Covid-19 infection on rates of premature birth, miscarriage and stillbirth in Chapter 1. Here I want to examine the effect of experiencing these events during a pandemic in terms of care received, alongside restrictions that were put in place around fertility treatment. How were women cared for when some of their worst fears had already come true?

Premature birth

We know that having a premature baby is often a time of considerable distress. Research has shown that feelings of shame, guilt and self-blame are common, with some mothers of babies in neonatal intensive care deliberately stopping themselves from bonding too deeply with their baby as a self-protective mechanism. Many parents are scared to touch their baby in case they hurt them.[1] Being separated from your baby and not being able to be with them in neonatal care can be phenomenally stressful for new mothers.[2] Unfortunately, it appeared that separation was just what happened for many new parents and babies during the pandemic. While most hospitals instigated visitor policies that significantly limited visiting on postnatal wards, some also appeared to apply this logic to the neonatal unit, in terms of mothers 'visiting' their premature baby.

Contact with premature babies is so important, both for the baby and parents. Lots of research has shown that being supported to hold your premature baby is associated with decreased maternal stress and anxiety and increased confidence.[3] Skin-to-skin contact is especially important for premature infants, helping to stabilise them and enhance the bond and connection between baby and parent.[4] Being able to talk, sing and read to your baby in neonatal care not only helps to further support that parent–infant bond, but also aids infant vocal development.[5] When parents regularly hold their premature baby in NICU, stress reactions in the infant decrease, alongside improvements in infant physical development. Babies were also more settled and happy to be held and examined.[6] These types of infant behaviour have been associated positively with cognitive, behavioural and educational outcomes in school-aged children.[7]

Breastmilk can be lifesaving for babies who are born very sick or prematurely. However, many babies who are in neonatal care have feeding challenges. Most do not develop a suck reflex until around 34 weeks, and mothers need to express breastmilk to feed them. This can be challenging at the best of times, but the difficulties can be exacerbated due to a premature or difficult birth, or the overwhelming stress of the situation. Conversely, being able to feed or provide milk for your premature baby can boost confidence and connection.[2] Notably, one of the things that can help most with expressing milk is being able to hold your baby or at least sit near them. Skin-to-skin increases the amount of milk produced, aided by increasing levels of oxytocin. Stress, although it does not inhibit milk production, can interfere with milk letdown.[8] A large multi-country study found that one of the strongest predictors of babies being exclusively breastfed on discharge from the neonatal unit was having a policy where parents could visit their baby as much as possible.[9]

So why on earth were so many mothers separated from their baby in neonatal care? In the previous chapters we saw how often mothers who had tested positive for Covid-19 were separated from their babies, with many infants sent to neonatal care even if they were not showing symptoms. There could arguably be some logic for this, even though it went against guidelines from the World Health Organization (and all the evidence that led to those guidelines). But what logic could justify separating healthy mothers from their babies?

When visitor policies were enacted across many healthcare systems due to Covid-19, mothers and babies got caught up in the changes. Somehow, some hospitals decided that a mother was a 'visitor' to her baby, rather than considering them a connected dyad. This meant that for many their experience of being able to care for their baby involved either not being able to see them at all (due to 'no visitor' restrictions) or having severely limited visiting restrictions. This went against all guidance. At no time was there a blanket policy in the UK that stated that mothers should not be able to be with their babies. Indeed, the Royal College of Paediatrics and Child Health (RCPCH),[10] British Association of Perinatal Medicine[11] and BLISS[12] the premature baby charity all stated that *'parental restrictions should be exercised only when absolutely necessary, as a temporary and proportionate response to a peak in viral transmission.'* Indeed both parents should be able to visit together, being treated as a family 'bubble'.

However, this often did not happen and restrictions were put in place. In one study 2,103 parents of a baby in special/intensive care from 56 countries completed a questionnaire about their experiences of visiting and caring for their baby.[13] Experiences varied significantly according to whether regulations in their country at the time required precautions, social distancing, complete lockdown or no concerns at all. Overall, 83% experienced some form of visiting restrictions. Specifically:

- Only 74% stated that mothers were allowed to visit, 56% fathers/partners, 3% siblings and 2% other family members.
- Only 32% of parents said that more than one parent could be present at once.
- 37% could visit freely, 18% several times a day, 19% once a day

and the remainder less frequently, with 15% unable to visit at all.

- 41% could stay for an unlimited duration but 30% were limited up to one hour.

In terms of contact with their baby:

- Only 10% had skin-to-skin contact within the first hour with 55% having to wait over a week.
- 30% were allowed to have as much skin-to-skin contact as they wanted, 27% once a day and 27% not at all.
- Just 79% were allowed to touch their baby in the incubator. Of these 53% could do so freely, 19% once a day and the rest less often.
- 35% had opportunity to sleep at the unit or a nearby special apartment. The remainder had to go home.
- 52% stated that no alternative forms of contact such as photos, live stream or videos were provided.

Justifiably, parents found this challenging – 71% found it more difficult to visit their baby and 61% found it more difficult to interact with and care for their baby. Almost a third of mothers and half of fathers had no involvement in their baby's day-to-day care (such as nappy changing) at all. The impact of this on maternal mental health was devastating. In one of the studies of women's pregnancy experience in the UK, one woman talked about her distress after giving birth to twins 12 weeks early. Her partner was sent straight home after the birth. Her babies were sent to neonatal care. She was placed alone in a side room, and eventually allowed to see her babies for just two hours. After that the hospital only allowed one parent to visit at a time.[14]

This was sadly not an isolated occurrence. In a study with mothers who had a baby in a neonatal unit in Italy, restrictions allowed one parent to visit for one hour per day. Understandably mothers were deeply affected by this experience, feeling sadness, anger and fear. They also felt lonely and distant from their partner who could not visit.[15] In another study in the US parents talked about how overwhelming and isolating the experience was, describing it as 'another level' of trauma on top of the already shocking impact of a baby being admitted to neonatal care.[16] In an Israeli study, feelings of helplessness were common among mothers separated from their baby, alongside fears they would contaminate them if they did visit.[17]

The long-term effects of all this could be significant. In a study with 231 parents with a baby in the NICU in the UK or USA, visiting restrictions meant that 27% could not take part in their baby's day-to-day care, 36% felt that breastfeeding had been negatively impacted and 41% were worried they had not bonded enough with their baby. Others struggled with wearing a face mask when in the unit, which 83% had to do (notably the RCPCH later advised that this was unnecessary); 34% were worried it was interfering with bonding and 21% felt it made interactions with staff less personal. Many felt that their overall experience was affected by only one parent being able to visit at a time, so they could not share the experience or lean on each other for support.[18]

Breastfeeding was damaged for many. In research that we conducted into parents' experiences of infant feeding during the pandemic (more on this in Chapter 6), we found that one in five mothers who had a baby admitted to neonatal care had their visiting stopped or restricted. This had a devastating impact on their ability to keep on breastfeeding. At the time of taking part in our study, 80% of those who had been restricted from seeing their baby had stopped breastfeeding, compared to less than 10% of those who had free access.[19] In a study in Turkey that examined human milk feeding in the NICU, rates dropped significantly at the start of the pandemic when guidelines and protocols were less clear and anxiety about the potential impact of Covid-19 on premature infants was greater. However, the authors noted that once clear guidelines were put in place to support breastfeeding and human milk feeding, rates increased again.[20]

Taking all this together, is it any wonder that rates of depression were high among parents with a baby in neonatal care during Covid-19? One study in the US involving 431 mothers and fathers of a NICU baby found that 33% of mothers and 17% of fathers had symptoms indicative of postnatal depression.[21]

Miscarriage and stillbirth

Around 10–15% of pregnancies end in miscarriage, defined as pregnancy loss before 20 weeks' gestation. Miscarriage is naturally associated with complex emotions, including feelings of grief and loss, shock, anger and anxiety around potential future pregnancies.[22] Understandably this can have significant effects on mental health. In one study exploring trauma symptoms in women experiencing moderate to high levels of grief after miscarriage, almost half had symptoms of post-traumatic stress.[23] Others experience clinically significant levels of anxiety or depression, which can be long-lasting. Many women still experience anxiety or depression up to three years after their loss – but we know this is likely an underestimate given how long we know memories of birth can last.[24] Ironically, one of the best things we know that can help parents through miscarriage is good social support, including the chance to talk about and process the loss with trusted friends and family – something that was of course severely affected by lockdowns.[25]

When I was researching the evidence for this chapter I was struck by how many papers had already emerged about the impact of Covid-19 on miscarriage and stillbirth. Notably, however, the vast majority of these papers were documenting miscarriage rates and potential influences on those rates. Of course this work is vitally important in helping protect future pregnancies. However, papers documenting women's experiences were starkly missing. I found one study that did explore the experiences of women who had a stillbirth or miscarriage during the pandemic. It was conducted in the US but open to women around the world, enabled by posting the links on websites such as Reddit.[26]

Overall 73 women took part, with three-quarters experiencing a miscarriage and a quarter a stillbirth. The authors identified three main ways in which women felt that their experiences had been affected by the pandemic. These were:

1. The lack of face-to-face support

When women had to attend face-to-face appointments or stay in hospital they typically had to do so alone, often waiting for hours in emergency situations. This meant that women were alone when they discovered that their baby had no heartbeat, or that there were complications. Many then went on to have procedures alone too. This understandably led to women feeling vulnerable and lonely, deprived of support when they needed it most – and ultimately very angry about the whole experience. Writer Caroline Criado-Perez, author of the bestselling feminist book *Invisible Women – Exposing Data Bias in a World Designed for Men* took to Twitter in December 2020 to document her own experience of miscarriage during a pandemic, detailing how traumatic and inhumane it was to leave women to face it alone.

On top of this, women were unable to meet family and friends face-to-face to break the news of their pregnancy loss. This further deprived them of their support network and the enhanced emotional support and physical contact they would have received. Women also found it traumatic having to make contact over phone or video call to tell people rather than being able to have a conversation face-to-face. Parents also could not reach out to other sources of support that they usually relied on, such as religious, sporting or social communities.

A lack of visitors at appointments or in hospital also affected family members. Partners could not see the ultrasound 'evidence' that their baby did not have a heartbeat. In the case of stillbirth women talked about how they were unable to have family attend the hospital to meet, hold and grieve their baby in person. In many cases family members were also unable to attend a funeral. The baby they were expecting to welcome into the family had effectively disappeared with no opportunity to say goodbye.

Finally, lockdown and not being able to meet people in each other's homes meant that recovering from miscarriage or stillbirth was even more distressing for parents who had older children. Some talked about how they had to come home from the hospital and continue caring for an older toddler or child who did not understand – without any possible break from someone else taking care of the child for a while.

2. Limited access to services

Covid regulations also changed the way in which many services around pregnancy loss were delivered. Although some services had to be face-to-face, those that could be delivered via video or phone call typically were. However, even when some appointments were in person, women talked about how procedures were delayed, prolonging their trauma. Although phone or video calls could relay practical information, women struggled with these when it came to counselling. Many local support groups were no longer running.

This was reflected in another study in which women talked about the distress of having to attend scans and appointments alone when they knew they had miscarried. Even at that point their partner was not allowed into the hospital to be with them, comfort them and help them process information. One woman described the distress of having to tell her partner over the phone that their baby had died, and then go on to receive treatment alone too.[14]

3. The emotional impact of losing a baby at this time

The isolation women experienced was recognised as having a negative impact on their mental health, making their feelings of grief and trauma feel stronger. Losing a baby would have been difficult at any time, but losing a baby when your support networks are severely curtailed was particularly traumatic.

Notably, some women talked about how the lack of connection with others meant that other people seem to forget about the pregnancy loss. One woman talked about not seeing anyone in person, so no one 'saw' the loss as such. Indeed, lockdown may have meant that family and friends had not seen 'evidence' of the pregnancy at all. Being away from others, such as working from home, would mean that the pregnancy would not have been so public. On the one hand this might have made intrusive questions less likely, but on the other hand women felt that it meant that their pregnancy did not exist in the eyes of those around them.

Another fear that women had was around trying to conceive another baby. This is always going to be a challenging decision after pregnancy loss, and many women report that their anxiety is greatly raised during the subsequent pregnancy. However, women were additionally worried about the possibility of losing another baby during the pandemic. This really goes to show the extent to which the pandemic affected their experience, over and above the pregnancy loss.

Fertility treatment

We've considered how the pandemic affected pregnancy and birth, but what about those who were hoping to become pregnant? Fertility treatment was rapidly halted at the start of the pandemic. In the UK the Human Fertilisation and Embryology Authority (HFEA), which regulates fertility treatment in the UK, ordered that all treatments should be halted by mid-April 2020, unless there was significant urgency, such as with cancer. In regions such as the US and Europe, restrictions were put in place in March, which had a range of consequences, from not being able to start treatment, to having to freeze fertilised eggs.[27]

We know that infertility can cause significant distress,

outside of the circumstances of the pandemic. Feelings of anger, depression, anxiety, a lack of control and stigma are all common. Social support is again an important aspect of coping with procedures, losses and all the stress involved.[28] Having choices taken away from you, with no details about when your treatment can resume and whether that will be too late is understandably deeply stressful, and stories started to emerge about the impact on couples undergoing fertility treatment.

A survey of 450 fertility clinic users (446 women and four men), showed a devastating impact of the pandemic on choices and decisions. The majority who responded (82%) had fertility tests or treatments postponed, whether they were publicly or self-funded. This naturally led to a whole host of negative emotions including stress, worry, frustration, anger and resentment. More than one in 10 felt that it had a significant impact on their mental health, feeling unable to cope with the decision at all. Indeed, 1% talked about suicidal ideation, feeling like they could not go on.[29]

Why did people find this disruption to treatment so challenging?

- Some felt that closures seemed too great a measure balanced against risk, particularly when there was no guidance saying that becoming pregnant would be dangerous.
- Others were worried about how the closures would affect their ability to get pregnant and have a family. With little notice about how long restrictions would last, and when treatment would be possible, some felt that time was running out. This was particularly difficult if couples had already experienced a lot of distress due to previously unsuccessful treatment or having to wait for a long time to start the process.
- Many felt left in the dark, waiting for updates that never came. After building what they felt were close relationships with clinics and staff, they felt abandoned or forgotten, as if

they were no longer important. This uncertainty led to some people becoming obsessed with the 'what ifs', and unable to focus on anything else.

- Others felt anger at those becoming pregnant naturally when their opportunity had been taken away. I can only imagine what it must have felt like to read headlines about how lockdowns would cause a 'baby boom', and hear jokes about lockdown pregnancies.

Some respondents were able to use the pause in treatment to try to focus on the future and improve their chances of success, such as having more time to lose weight, become more physically active or to address any other health needs. Others felt that there was a 'silver lining', finding that being forced to take a break allowed them to process emotions between cycles, or to come to terms with having to adapt treatments such as receiving donor eggs.

In another study of fertility patients in Israel who had their treatment stopped, similar reactions were reported. Women described how they felt angry (23%), helpless (61%), sad (64%) and distressed (50%). However, again a small proportion (9%) felt a sense of relief. These findings were replicated in studies around the world, with one US-based study finding that 22% of fertility patients felt that withdrawal of treatment felt equivalent to losing a child.[30]

In one study that examined rates of symptoms of anxiety and depression among fertility patients, 21% of women and 13% of men exhibited clinically significant levels of depression and 24% of women and 18% of men exhibited clinically significant levels of anxiety. Of those, 8% of women and 6% of men exhibited clinically significant levels of both. Rates were higher among those suffering female or male-factor fertility. Overall 46% of women with female-factor fertility experienced anxiety or depression, compared to 21% of those without. In men 29% with male-factor fertility experienced anxiety or depression compared to 16% without.[31]

Women showed significant splits in how necessary they felt

that suspension of services was. Around half did not feel that suspension was justified at all, with the remainder feeling that it was important for patients' own health (31%), risks of becoming pregnant during Covid-19 (28%), the impact of the pandemic on health resources (17%) and the health and availability of healthcare providers (8%). Notably those who felt it was justified had significantly higher anxiety levels than those who did not. Around three-quarters wished that fertility treatment could restart. Those who didn't want treatment to restart expressed fears around infection and safety, not wanting to give birth during a pandemic and lockdown and financial concerns.[32]

A Canadian study of women and men who were attending a fertility clinic found that 43% disagreed with guidelines to stop treatment, with 82% willing to resume treatments if it were possible. This shows the significance of the situation – presumably some believed that guidelines were logical, but would still take the perceived risk if it meant resuming treatment. Many of those who disagreed with suspension guidelines viewed fertility treatment as an essential medical treatment, exacerbated by the time-sensitive nature for many of those undergoing it. Similar data emerged in the US study, with 86% stating that they would prefer to be able to make an informed decision in conversation with their doctor, and 52% stating they would definitely start a new cycle if possible (with a further 21% unsure).[30]

Those who would not be willing to recommence treatment had greater anxieties about the risks of Covid-19. Many in this group saw a need to prioritise saving lives due to Covid-19, or to not take away PPE when they believed it was in shortage. Others were simply scared of contracting Covid-19 when pregnant.[33]

We must make sure we look at the bigger picture: balancing risk from Covid-19 against the need for sensitive care around pregnancy complications. Separating mother and baby without clear reason is inhumane and many parents will need support to process their traumatic experiences during this time.

5

POSTNATAL CARE DURING THE PANDEMIC

POSTNATAL CARE
DURING THE PANDEMIC

The perinatal period is a time of huge change, particularly for first-time parents who are transitioning into a new role as parents. Although this can be a time of celebration and joy, the intense needs of newborn babies, combined with the shock of the intensity of early parenting, can leave new parents feeling overwhelmed and exhausted.[1] With many new parents having little prior experience of caring for newborn babies, misconceptions about normal baby behaviour, such as how often babies wake and feed, are common and can lead to anxiety that something is wrong.[2]

In many cultures around the world, the needs of new parents are recognised far more than they are in westernised countries such as the UK. A greater sense of community and connection means that new mothers are not caring for their babies in isolation or without information and support. However, in the UK many new parents are forced to cope with the transition to parenthood without the support of such a connected community around them.[3] Many new parents live a considerable distance from family and rather than being supported during the newborn period, they instead face isolation and loneliness.[4]

The impact of this shock, isolation and inexperience can have a significant negative impact on parental wellbeing.[5] It can also affect how well equipped parents are to care for their baby, in terms of understanding what is normal and where they need further attention and support. To combat this, a programme of postnatal care has been established in the UK and other similar countries that is designed to support infant health and development and the mental health and wellbeing of new parents. In England the Healthy Child Programme sets out a series of support visits that are mandatory for health visitors to offer, including an antenatal contact, post-birth check, and health and development checks at 6–8 weeks, 9 months and 2–2.5 years. Alongside this a programme of vaccination, baby weighing, baby development, mental health and support for families should be available.[6]

We know that consistent support is really important during the postnatal period. A systematic review of research into what works best in terms of the delivery of postnatal support found that the best outcomes for maternal wellbeing were associated with regular, consistent and face-to-face support at home in the first six weeks after birth. Although support around practical elements of infant care was important, women most valued care that was focused on psychological and social support.[7] Indeed, postnatal programmes that help support parental wellbeing, providing a sense of reassurance and community, are valued by new parents.[8]

Unfortunately, even before the pandemic hit, postnatal care services in the UK were being cut. Termed the 'Cinderella service' of maternity care, concerns have been raised over the past decade over its provision, with the Chief Medical Officer for England declaring it 'not fit for purpose' back in 2014.[9]

Changes to health visiting due to the pandemic

The pandemic dramatically affected health visiting (and therefore the support that new families received) in three main ways. First, the needs of new parents vastly increased. Second, redeployment of health visitors into Covid-19 and other nursing roles reduced the workforce. Third, significant reductions in face-to-face appointments affected the quality of the care delivered and received. The combination of these three key factors led to the Institute of Health Visiting describing services as being at 'breaking point',[10] and has had a huge impact on parents' experiences, particularly in terms of support with feeding, mental health and baby development – all of which we will look at separately in the next three chapters.

The impact of the pandemic on the delivery of health visiting services has been clearly documented. Every year the Institute of Health Visiting publishes a report on the work, experiences and needs of health visitors working in England. The seventh annual *State of Health Visiting in England* report for 2020 included the impact of the Covid-19 pandemic on health visiting services. The report included the views of 862 health visitors in England, finding that compared to two years earlier:[11]

- **82% felt that they had seen an increase in domestic violence**
- **81% an increase in perinatal mental illness**
- **81% an increase in family poverty**
- **76% an increase in food bank use**
- **75% an increase in speech/communication delay**
- **61% an increase in child neglect**
- **45% an increase in families struggling with substance abuse**

Likewise, in a survey of 740 health visitors in England by researchers at University College London, many were worried about how vulnerable children were being protected. In terms of the proportion concerned about different aspects:[12]

- **96% were concerned about domestic violence and abuse**
- **92% about parental mental health conditions**
- **86% about safeguarding**
- **82% about child neglect**
- **84% about children's growth**
- **79% about children's development**
- **75% about breastfeeding**

- 63% about the lack of health check-ups
- 49% about childhood vaccination uptake

These fears were sadly not unfounded. In November 2020 Amanda Spielman, chief inspector of Ofsted, referred to the pandemic and lockdown as causing a 'pressure cooker' for families with young children, with councils reporting a rise of 20% in incidents of serious harm to children under one. Compared to data from the previous year, a particular rise had been seen in serious incident notifications for children under one, with 40% of all cases involving a child of this age. Although this figure does include accidents, more than half of these cases were non-accidental, including eight deaths.

What caused this? Spielman referred to the same causes we have already looked at throughout this book – the combination of isolation, a loss of family support, financial hardship and loss of employment coming together to form a 'toxic mix' for families who were already vulnerable and struggling with mental health issues, substance misuse and poverty.[13]

These concerns were replicated in other data. In a study comparing the incidence of suspected abusive head trauma among children at one hospital during the first month of lockdown, to the rate over the last three years, a significant increase in trauma was found. During this period 10 children, with an average age of around six months were seen, whereas the average figure per month in the previous years was 0.67. This represented an increase of 1493%. The authors were concerned that this was an under-representation of how many children were actually exposed to head injuries due to the general low attendance at A&E at the time.[14]

Major spikes in domestic abuse cases were also seen. Although these are often reported between adult couples, abuse in the home can clearly affect children too. Research shows that up to two-thirds of children living in homes where domestic abuse occurs are also victims of abuse. Parents who are themselves abused are at increased risk of neglecting their children or adopting an abusive parenting style. Similar increases were seen in other countries. In one study in the US, the Childhelp National Child Abuse Hotline reported 31% more calls in March 2020 than the previous March. Lockdown of course exacerbated proximity to abuse. In one US study, 79% of those who contacted a sexual assault hotline were living with their abuser.[15]

The impact of health visitor redeployment

At the start of the pandemic, when no one knew how long it would all last, or the severity of pressure on health services that would result, significant numbers of health visitors were redeployed into other nursing roles – either on Covid-19 wards or to support other wards where staff had been moved. The *State of Health Visiting in England* report found that 20% of health visitors surveyed had been redeployed, with 20% also stating that over 50% of health visitors in their team had been redeployed.

In the research led by University College London examining the impact of the first lockdown on health visiting services,[12] it was found that:

- 61% of health visitors reported that someone from their team had been redeployed
- Managers of health visitors reported up to 80% of their team being redeployed
- 10% of managers reported over 50% of their team being redeployed

In a follow-up report using freedom of information requests,[16] the UCL team examined the extent of redeployment again. They found that during the first wave of the lockdown:

- 66% of local authorities in England redeployed at least one member of the health visiting team
- Redeployment numbers ranged from 0–63% of teams
- 11% of local authorities redeployed 25% or more of their teams
- Average duration of redeployment was 2.2 months
- 73% of local authorities who redeployed staff continued to do so after June 2020 when it was advised not to do so

Obviously the number of families needing health visitor care did not reduce. Whereas the recommended maximum caseload per health visitor is 250 children under five (which still seems like an awful lot to me), in the *State of Health Visiting in England* report 65% of health visitors surveyed had caseloads 20% greater than that, with 29% having an increase of two-thirds, and 12% supporting caseloads double that size.

Of course when workload is increased/staffing is reduced, the services offered also have to reduce. When limited time is available, staff need to focus on the most urgent cases, leaving those in less serious situations to perhaps not receive the care that they need, or dropping non-urgent care. Indeed, two-thirds of health visitors reported that they had limited capacity to deliver prevention/early intervention support, with their time focused predominantly on safeguarding.

The consequences for care are clear. The *State of Health Visiting in England* report found that just 17% of health visitors were able to offer all families in their care the 9–12 month review, dropping to 10% for the two-year review. This came on the back of a steady decline in health visiting numbers over the past five years. One report found that compared to 2015 there are almost one-third fewer health visitors in post – even before you add in the impact of the pandemic.[17]

Simultaneously, other services were also being reduced. Over 90% of health visitors reported a reduction in children's centre services and children's social services, meaning that even more of a burden fell upon health visiting. This led to some health visitors feeling that they had to respond to at-risk families for whom other services would usually have been involved, again further reducing the time they could spend on other less immediately urgent issues.

Understandably the workload had a knock-on impact on the stress levels and mental health of staff. In the UCL report 68% reported that their stress levels had increased, 70% were working longer hours and a third felt that they would leave the profession if they could. Likewise, in the *State of Health Visiting in England* report:

- **75% reported increased stress**
- **70% were working longer hours**
- **69% felt worried, tense and anxious**
- **51% reported that their sleep was affected**
- **40% were experiencing low mood due to work-related stress**

As well as there being pressure on health visitors delivering services, there was also an impact on the support health visitors themselves were receiving. Overall half of health visitors reported that they had no access to clinical supervision, with just one in five saying they had received 'restorative supervision', which is designed to help health professionals process the complex and often distressing nature of their work.

Impact on service delivery

As with antenatal care, the pandemic impacted on service delivery in two main ways – which services were allowed to continue, and which services were able to continue due to reduced staffing. At the start of the first wave of the pandemic NHS England and NHS Improvement published guidelines on 1 April that prevented much health visiting support from going ahead. All services were told to stop apart from the antenatal contact, new baby visits and visits for vulnerable families (although these had to be assessed on a case-by-case basis). Where possible contacts were to be virtual, using video or telephone calls. Where face-to-face care was needed, PPE had to be worn.

Thankfully, as the pandemic continued and the consequences for new families were recognised, some other services were restarted. At the beginning of June 2020 health visiting services were given the go-ahead to recommence fully, alongside services such as community paediatrics and school nursing.[18] However, due to the other issues surrounding the pandemic such as redeployment, staff sickness and the need for social distancing, some elements of services had to be prioritised, such as those for mental health or vulnerable families.

Examination of the contacts that did go ahead shows that disruption to services continued. In the *State of Health Visiting in England* report, health visitors were asked whether they had been able to offer the five mandatory health and development checks in the Healthy Child Programme to all families during the pandemic. Overall:

- **35% had offered all families an antenatal visit**
- **79% a new birth visit**
- **67% a 6–8 week check**
- **17% a 9–12 month check**
- **10% a 2–2.5 year check**

Some appointments were conducted by community nursery nurses or family support workers, despite Public Health England guidance that these should be delivered by health visitors. It is not clear in the report how many of these took place face-to-face or via video/phone call, but looking at similar data from the UCL study of which contacts occurred during the first lockdown, just

16% of health visitors surveyed reported carrying out face-to-face antenatal visits, 47% new birth visits and 62% safeguarding visits. Instead, lots of contacts occurred by phone. Likewise, in the *Babies in Lockdown* report only 11% of parents of under-twos reported having seen a health visitor face-to-face during the early months of the pandemic. Anecdotally, although in some areas contacts have been reinstated, I have also received many messages from parents who haven't seen a health visitor or other health professional for a very long time, some since the start of the pandemic.

Additionally, many parents were confused about whether face-to-face support would be offered and where. In Ireland, women are typically visited at home by a public health nurse within 72 hours of returning home from hospital. In one interview study with new mothers, many described how they did not receive this visit at home, instead having to take their newborn baby out to their local health centre to see the public health nurse. A phone call appointment was offered first to cover aspects that didn't need face-to-face care. This presented issues with the logistics of getting to the centre, the exhaustion and pain of doing so if recovering from a difficult birth, and fear of transmission of Covid-19. Some of the women in the study highlighted how communication about this change was not clear, with some having to make several phone calls to work out whether someone was coming or where they had to go.[19]

Overall it was recommended that virtual contacts should still take place where possible, although the guidance did state that '*Face-to-face contacts should be prioritised for families who are not known to services to mitigate known limitations of virtual contacts and support effective assessment of needs/ risks*'.[18] Reflecting on the efficacy of providing health visiting support via video call, in the *State of Health Visiting in England* report, 89% of health visitors surveyed felt that video contacts were not as effective at identifying the needs of parents or encouraging them to disclose issues as face-to-face appointments. This was particularly true when sensitive topics needed to be discussed. Two-thirds of health visitors felt that video contact was inappropriate when families needed support with things like perinatal mental health, rising to 88% for issues such as safeguarding, domestic abuse and substance misuse. However, most felt that they worked well if simple or quick advice was needed.

Research into how useful telephone calls can be in supporting health is mixed. Some studies show that it can be a useful and efficient form of support if queries are simple, which reflects the views of health visitors in the *State of Health Visiting in England* survey. However, for more complex issues, a negative impact is often seen. People can be reluctant to talk about concerns over the phone, with fewer disclosures of information and shorter discussions when they do arise.[20]

This certainly seemed to be the experience of many parents. In one interview study with pregnant and postnatal women, many talked about how the relative absence of health visitors or lack of emotional connection in phone or video calls impacted negatively on their wellbeing.[21] They felt unable to raise serious issues, and found it difficult to check in with small concerns about their baby's health or wellbeing, or how they themselves were recovering and coping. Although advice could be given by phone, many wanted the reassurance of their baby actually being seen in person to check that things were fine. Others simply missed that human connection and the validation of someone saying 'you're doing a great job'.

Although face-to-face appointments should have been available when needed, some women found themselves only able to access phone call support for physical issues after birth. In the *Babies in Lockdown* report, a new mother describes how she was worried about her episiotomy stitches. She was told that she would need to contact the GP to receive antibiotics, but in order to be 'diagnosed' she would have to take photos of her vulva and send them to a generic GP practice email address. This naturally felt like a complete invasion of her privacy. This was echoed in another study in Washington with women finding it really difficult to talk about and convey their symptoms and experience of post-birth pain over a video or phone call.[22] Others found that when they tried to seek telephone support for physical issues such as episiotomy or wound pain, they felt that their symptoms were ignored or misinterpreted without a proper examination. For many women their six-week postnatal check was simply cancelled.[23]

Video calls also require the use of technology and a stable internet connection, which pushes families from more deprived backgrounds further into disadvantage. One study with nurses working at a Maternal, Infant, and Early Childhood Home Visiting service in Florida found that while video calls worked well with some families, they raised a number of issues around internet connectivity, cost and a lack of suitable devices.[24] Many ended up switching off video to get a better connection, but this of course meant that all visual interaction was lost, reducing emotional connection and meaning that nurses could not assess parent–infant relationships. Other families simply did not have the digital skills to conduct video calls in an effective way.

When face-to-face contact did go ahead, it was often nothing like the usual contacts, with reductions in time spent in the home and a focus on practical checks only, alongside social distancing and wearing of PPE. In terms of PPE, one example from the 'health for under-fives' website[25] stated that:

'When a member of the Health Visiting team visits you, they will be wearing some or all of the following before entering your home: an apron, gloves, a face mask, goggles or a visor... When the health professional leaves your home they will remove all PPE and put it in a black bin bag for you to dispose of in your household waste'.

Of course PPE was put in place to reduce potential transmission and to protect both health professionals and parents. However, it had a subsequent impact on the professional–parent relationship. Health visiting is based around these relationships, often in the home setting. It is about listening and giving guidance rather than a 'clinical' medical appointment. How easy would it be for a new mother in the depths of postnatal depression to open up to someone sat on the other side of the room wearing goggles?

What about families who are more vulnerable?

The postnatal period can be tough enough without support when you are in a stable living situation. But what happened to families who were already more vulnerable and disrupted? For those families who were really struggling, the impacts of lockdown were significant. The closure of children's centres meant that they had less contact with staff who could support them. Virtual communication (which was often via phone due to connectivity issues) meant that harms could go unseen, with it being more difficult to physically assess child wellbeing. The excuse of 'staying safe' could be used to avoid contact with professionals. Suspension of birth registration meant that babies were going unseen and not receiving post-birth visits. This all happened against a backdrop of the exacerbation of existing stressors such as poverty, food insecurity, mental health issues, domestic violence and substance misuse.[26]

At the start of the pandemic there were approximately 135,000 children living in temporary accommodation in the UK. Those classed in official figures were typically based in hostels or bed and breakfast accommodation, but many other families outside of the system are staying with relatives or friends without a formal home of their own.[27] There is considerable evidence that while these temporary living circumstances place a roof over families' heads, they do not provide optimal living conditions for young children. Families can be placed in accommodation out of their local area. Often accommodation is damp, unsafe or overcrowded, typically with shared kitchen and bathroom facilities. Many families live in one room with little space or opportunity for children to play.[28]

The impact on families living in these circumstances during Covid-19 was devastating.[29] Lockdown, social distancing and isolation were distressing enough for families living in their own accommodation. However, a number of different aspects of temporary accommodation increased the trauma for families. These included:

- Shared kitchen and bathroom facilities increasing risk of transmission
- Isolation or simply lockdown in one overcrowded room
- One-room accommodation making isolating impossible for those who were unwell with Covid-19
- Enforced stay-at-home legislation meaning that issues such as shared accommodation with those with drug or alcohol problems or behavioural issues becoming more constant
- No internet connection exacerbating issues
- The exhaustion of trying to entertain bored children who have few toys or play opportunities
- Exacerbation of parental mental health issues, substance misuse and simply reduced sleep, making responsive, child-centred care feel like an impossibility

Some families have been able to move to more suitable accommodation, but this also had a negative impact in other ways:

- Losing social connections at a time where any connection felt important
- Services closing that helped individuals during moves such

as grant offices and charity shops
- **Difficulties registering with a new GP**

One measure to try to better support families living in these conditions was the introduction of specialist health visiting posts specifically for homeless families. However, this became even more challenging during lockdown. Issues identified by one specialist health visitor included:

- **Not being able to find families**
- **A lack of internet connection or devices to do video calls**
- **Language and communication barriers making phone or virtual calls difficult**
- **Rooms so small that social distancing during appointments is impossible**

Moving forward

Eventually the impact of the pandemic on postnatal care was recognised, albeit it too late for those affected in the first lockdown. In October 2020 NHS England's chief nurse Ruth May, Professor Viv Bennett, chief nurse at Public Health England, and Councillor Ian Hudspeth from the Local Government Association published a letter highlighting the severity of the impact of reducing health visiting services.[30] They referred to health visiting as a 'front line service' and stated that:

'It is now known that the indirect impact of Covid-19 has been significant for pregnant women, children, young people and families. There have been increases in safeguarding concerns, domestic abuse, child and maternal mental health problems as well as lost learning time for all children, impacting on outcomes for safety and wellbeing.

Sustaining support for families needs to be a priority if

short and long term harms are to be prevented, identified and mitigated. Therefore, we advise that professionals supporting children and families, such as health visitors, school nurses, designated safeguarding officers and nurses supporting children with special educational needs should not be redeployed to other services and should be supported to provide services through pregnancy, early years (0–19) and to the most vulnerable families'.

The report was welcomed by the Institute of Health Visiting, with Dr Cheryll Adams, executive director, stating that she was:

'pleased and relieved that the chief nurses and LGA have supported our campaign for health visitors not to be redeployed again... This profession has its own front line and infants and their families have never needed them more than they do at the moment.'

This was echoed by Alison Morton, deputy executive director at the Institute of Health Visiting:[31]

'Babies and young children were largely invisible in the first wave of the government's emergency plans... With a growing body of evidence, we now know that many children are being harmed by the secondary impact of the pandemic and we cannot knowingly overlook their needs again, as we live with the virus for the foreseeable future.'

It is clear that the changes to health visiting services during the pandemic negatively affected the care given to new parents and the health and wellbeing of them and their babies. Alongside the broader impacts of lockdown and social isolation, over the next three chapters we will consider how infant feeding, mental health and baby health and development were specifically affected.

6

EXPERIENCES OF INFANT FEEDING DURING THE PANDMEIC

EXPERIENCES OF INFANT FEEDING DURING THE PANDEMIC

Eighteen months on from the initial lockdown in the UK, it is clear that the pandemic and subsequent lockdowns had an impact on women's experiences of feeding their baby – whether they were breast or bottle-feeding. However, as with many experiences during the pandemic the effects appeared to be starkly different for individual families. While some on one level appeared to thrive, others were far more negatively affected, with many stopping breastfeeding before they were ready, due to scaremongering in the press about the supposed safety of breastfeeding, and the impact of the lockdown and social distancing on breastfeeding support.

Families who were formula feeding were not exempt from this chaos. Panic-buying and hoarding temporarily affected the formula supply chain in some supermarkets and ignited fears about how babies would be fed. Babies under six months old who are not breastfed or receiving human milk must be given formula milk. There is no alternative, as there is with other foods, and anxieties were running high. Some tried to exploit this by selling milks online at extortionate prices.[1]

Dr Natalie Shenker and I undertook a piece of research exploring the experiences of mothers in the UK who were breastfeeding during the first lockdown. We collected data in May–June 2020, exploring the experiences of those who were already breastfeeding before lockdown and those who gave birth during it. Over 1,200 mothers took part. It was clear that although some mothers were able to continue breastfeeding exclusively, those who had stopped or introduced formula had done so fairly rapidly. The average time of stopping was when their baby was just three weeks old, with formula often being introduced by the second week.[2] Similar data emerged in the *Babies in Lockdown* study[3] and in research in other countries such as the US[4], Ireland[5], and Italy.[6]

Most critical for me was the depressing finding in our study that just 13.5% of those who had stopped breastfeeding felt ready to do so. Most had planned to breastfeed for longer. Likewise, of those mothers who had started mixed feeding, over 80% said they had never planned to do so or had thought they might when their baby was much older. Similarly in the *Babies in Lockdown* report 53% of those using formula milk had not planned to do so.[3] So what went wrong?

Contaminated breastmilk?

The one thing we can pretty much all agree – whatever your stance on the pandemic and the safety measures – is the negative impact of the fearmongering press that increasingly spread unfounded rumours about how and where Covid-19 could be transmitted. If you could imagine something as a potential means of transmission, no matter how implausible, the press had already written six different articles on it and found someone somewhere who had supposedly contracted Covid-19 in this way (and had a sad face photo taken for a tabloid newspaper).

Sadly, breastfeeding and human milk were not exempt from this approach. In the early weeks of lockdown in the UK and many other countries, headlines and rumours spread in the press and on social media suggesting that the virus could be spread through breastmilk or breastfeeding. At the time, as Covid-19 was a novel pathogen, we didn't have any data to prove this wrong. How do you prove the uniform absence of something? Not rapidly, that's for sure. Scientists were asking questions and as usual a question was interpreted as a 'potential threat' and soon stories were abounding about this 'risk'.

All this fearmongering had an impact. Unfortunately, the American Academy of Pediatrics initially recommended separating mother and baby in case of suspected infection,[7] guidance that thankfully has since changed to keep them together.[8] As we saw in Chapter 3 the World Health Organization quickly stated that breastfeeding should continue even when mothers had tested positive for Covid-19 (albeit with hygiene measures such as masks). The risk to babies from Covid-19 was seen as so low, and the protection of breastfeeding so high, that even with a potential transmission risk breastfeeding was still to be encouraged and supported.[9]

However, despite organisations in the UK rapidly putting out statements affirming that mothers and babies should remain together and breastfeeding should be encouraged, not all similar health bodies around the world followed that lead. Globally mothers and babies were routinely separated at some point during the pandemic in China, Malaysia, the Philippines, Indonesia and more, with breastmilk substitutes sometimes recommended.[10] These recommendations had an impact in other countries. Stories quickly spread across global online media, increasing fear and leading to even more separations, and mothers avoiding breastfeeding 'just in case'.

At the time we were conducting our research there was no evidence of transmission of Covid into breastmilk, just as studies of previous outbreaks had shown no transfer of viruses such as Middle East respiratory virus (MERS) or SARS. And time proved this right. As I write now there have been a number of published papers and showing no transmission of the virus into breastmilk. Although there have been a small number of case studies that have identified very low number of tiny viral fragments in samples of breastmilk expressed by symptomatic women,[11] this is miles away from the virus actually being present to be transferred to and infect a baby. Indeed, the World Health Organization conducted a systematic review of these types of reports, concluding that none of them had actually identified intact viral particles, or shown that these particles were actually capable of infecting anyone.[12]

There were also queries raised about the methodology of some of these studies. For example, a symptomatic mother expressing her milk might accidentally transfer the virus to the milk during or after expressing, either on her hands or from coughing. And actually as noted in Chapter 3 the opposite was also found: a case study in Australia of a symptomatic mother who was careful with handwashing and mask wearing showed that she did not pass the virus to her baby despite frequent feeding and contact.[13]

Of course, it seems that whenever we talk about potential harms of breastfeeding, we never seem to consider the potential harms of *not* breastfeeding and how these weigh up overall. Given the low individual risk of Covid-19 to infants even if they did contract it, and the likelihood of the mother already having passed it on if she was going to, the case for not breastfeeding was weak as it was. But apparently this risk was the only part visible to hospitals and health professionals recommending (or dictating) separation. As is so often the case, the copious evidence that demonstrates the long-term health protection offered by breastfeeding, to mother and baby, was not considered.[14] Certainly the significant and long-lasting emotional implications of not being able to breastfeed were ignored.[15]

In our research we asked mothers about their perceptions of the messaging around the safety of breastfeeding. We found that over a fifth of mothers who stopped breastfeeding during lockdown attributed their decision in part to fears about the safety of breastfeeding, with 6.5% stopping after they developed symptoms of the virus (although not always with a positive test). These anxieties were also present in those who continued breastfeeding. Overall, almost one in six mothers said they were anxious about the possibility of infecting their baby through breastfeeding, although most felt that their fears had eased slightly as the pandemic went on.

Similar concerns have been reported in studies in other countries. In Australia, 10% of mothers seeking support from the Australian Breastfeeding Association raised concerns over safety.[16] In the US, where many mothers return to work within weeks of giving birth due to a lack of maternity leave, one study found that mothers were particularly anxious about the safety of expressing and storing milk for their baby. They were concerned that all the different steps involved in the process, such as storage and transport, could introduce infection into their milk.[17]

What was particularly concerning was that 4% of mothers reported that they were told by a health professional that breastfeeding might not be safe during the pandemic, with 3% being told they would not be allowed to breastfeed if they had any symptoms. One in six also reported that they were told they might have to wear a mask when feeding their baby, even if they didn't have any symptoms. This may seem like a reassuringly small percentage of women, but spread out over a larger population this could mean that inaccurate messaging was reaching many thousands of women. Indeed, we found that those who had stopped breastfeeding were significantly more likely to have been told by a health professional that it was unsafe or would not be allowed.

Social media was also recognised as spreading distressing messages. Although many positive and accurate messages about supporting breastfeeding were shared on social media, misleading and inaccurate messages emerged too.[18] In our study, over a fifth of mothers reported seeing articles online that said breastfeeding was not safe, with 10% being forwarded or told about such articles by concerned family and friends. We know that friends and family can have a big influence on whether a mother feels comfortable or able to continue breastfeeding. Additional fearmongering, anxieties or pressure to stop breastfeeding may well have had an impact. As one mother in our research noted: '*I wanted to carry on but my partner was so anxious about our baby due to things he had read that in the end I agreed to cut things short and give formula instead*'.

These media stories and rumours had a knock-on effect beyond directly affecting the decision to continue breastfeeding. One in three mothers in our survey did not contact a health professional when they were experiencing breastfeeding difficulties because of worries about contracting the virus or that the health system was overloaded and falling apart. We have already seen in previous chapters how anxiety prevented mothers from contacting health professionals during birth and the postnatal period. Breastfeeding support was no different. This was also echoed in another study with pregnant and new mothers at the time. Almost two-thirds of mothers said they would be concerned if they needed to see a health professional face-to-face for support. Sadly, as might be predicted, not contacting a health professional when a problem arose was associated with stopping breastfeeding early.[19]

The impact of lockdown on access to breastfeeding support

In our research we also explored how the pandemic and lockdown affected the support women had received. When lockdown hit, face-to-face breastfeeding support was withdrawn in many areas, although in some places it did appear to remain possible to access face-to-face support in some situations. Everything had to be moved online or done via phone call. Peer support groups, a vital connection and source of support for many breastfeeding mothers,[20] were cancelled and moved online. Given that we know that breastfeeding support, particularly regular, consistent and face-to-face support, is key to enabling more mothers to breastfeed for longer,[21] the potential implications of this were huge.

To try to remain positive… it wasn't all bad. Overall, around 40% of mothers felt they did receive sufficient practical support with breastfeeding from health professionals, and 36% felt they received enough emotional support (though the obvious flip side of these statistics is that many did not). Indeed, over two-thirds felt that lockdown had led to a reduction in the available breastfeeding support. Unsurprisingly, those who were still breastfeeding felt more supported than those who had stopped. We also found that access to support was not equal. We found that women with higher levels of education and from White backgrounds were more likely to report that they had accessed enough support and that it was high quality and met their needs. Women from Black, Asian and minority ethnic backgrounds were less likely to feel they had received sufficient practical support compared to those from White backgrounds.

The *Babies in Lockdown* report painted a similar picture. Many mothers did manage to start and continue breastfeeding, but half of those who were using formula had not planned to do so, with a quarter feeling that they did not get the breastfeeding support that they needed.[3] And in *The Covid-19 New Mum Study* many breastfeeding women reported a lack of face-to-face support, which particularly affected them when they were experiencing complications. Many could not get the support they needed and turned to formula milk instead.[22] Similar data emerged from the US, with a switch to telehealth being given as a main reason for breastfeeding cessation or introduction of formula milk.[4]

In our research we asked women who had stopped breastfeeding what had led to that decision. The usual suspects that we see all the time outside of the pandemic were there. Common reasons included issues with latch, pain, insufficient milk and exhaustion. But we then asked whether they felt that the pandemic had directly affected these issues. Unsurprisingly, most women who had stopped breastfeeding felt that it had. Over 70% attributed a lack of face-to-face support to not being able to continue. Indeed, 85% of those who had been unable to continue breastfeeding felt that reduced support due to the regulations was a core issue. But something was also stopping women from reaching out for support. Overall, of those who needed support, just 43% contacted a health professional and 42% contacted a breastfeeding organisation.

What went so wrong?

We know that although breastfeeding might be the biologically 'normal' way that mammals have always fed their babies, it isn't always easy or straightforward. Many women in the UK want to breastfeed but experience challenges and complications that lead them to stop breastfeeding before they are ready.[23] Compared to other countries things are particularly challenging within our UK culture and we have some of the lowest breastfeeding rates in the world.[24]

Given that historically we have evolved as mammals to feed our babies human milk, why has it become so complicated? In a nutshell, the invention of formula milk at the end of the 19th century was on the one hand beneficial for babies who could not receive breastmilk, but on the other hand caused immeasurable harm to breastfeeding. The invention led to the creation of the formula milk industry, which was intent on making a profit from the product, and ultimately from new families.

Formula use expanded rapidly, particularly within hospital and medical settings where it was promoted as equal to or even better than breastmilk. By the 1950s many doctors and paediatricians caring for babies and birthing women were strong proponents of formula milk, viewing it as something that could be measured, fed to babies by someone else and provided everything a baby needed. Endorsement led to rapidly falling breastfeeding rates and a generation of breastfeeding knowledge and experience was lost. Formula feeding became normalised and breastfeeding became something that was not commonly seen, accepted or understood.

Fast forward a few decades and increasing amounts of research showed that at a population level, breastfeeding protected the health of both babies and mothers, having significant positive impacts on healthcare resources and costs. Public health organisations realised the importance of promoting breastfeeding, but unfortunately significant damage had been done. Whereas in previous generations we would have learnt about breastfeeding from seeing it all around us, and our families and communities would have held knowledge on how to support it, much of this had gone. Breastfeeding was promoted, but without this support, rates were slow to rise.[25]

This meant that support for breastfeeding often had to be provided to families 'externally', by health professionals, specialists and peer supporters (other women who had experience of breastfeeding their own baby). Research has now shown just how important that support can be. A recent review of evidence found that where breastfeeding education and support was provided by trained and experienced professionals and peer supporters, breastfeeding rates increased. The best outcomes came from consistent and regular support, particularly delivered face-to-face, throughout the postnatal period.

This support was also valued by mothers. In particular support that combined both practical elements such as help with positioning and attachment, alongside emotional support and encouragement, was seen as important. Time was also an important element: where health professionals could simply spend time sitting and chatting to mothers, offering advice and reassurance where needed, maternal confidence increased. Peer supporters played a large role in this, providing practical tips, a feeling of breastfeeding being 'normal', and encouraging a feeling of community support and reassurance.

It's hardly rocket science to understand where this all went wrong in the pandemic. In the first wave and subsequent lockdown, much of the face-to-face support women relied on disappeared almost overnight. Local breastfeeding peer support groups were not allowed to meet, and limits were also placed on health professionals.[26]

Moving support online – the positives

With the rapid change in circumstances, many breastfeeding organisations, breastfeeding specialists and lactation consultants moved mountains to adapt their support to online formats as much as was feasibly possible. Phone, email and video support was used, including online peer support groups. As part of our research we explored what types of support families were using and what for.

When mothers accessed online breastfeeding support from charity organisations, the vast majority found it useful and supportive in helping answer their queries and overcome difficulties. Queries included all the usual concerns around milk supply, pain, frequency of feeding and infections. This echoed similar research exploring the reasons why mothers contacted the Australian Breastfeeding Association during lockdown.[16] Clearly these charity organisations were playing a major role in fielding queries and concerns and supporting mothers to breastfeed through deeply challenging circumstances.

We also looked at how many women found different sources useful. Overall, 86% found one-to-one video calls useful, 84% found social media posts useful, 75% found group video calls useful and 70% found text messages useful. Overall, 98% agreed that online support was useful during the pandemic, with 81% wanting it to remain as an option when face-to-face meeting was possible again. However, notably very few mothers would have been happy for it to replace face-to-face support altogether.

How was online support seen as useful? Mainly for the

convenience. It was rapid, didn't require going anywhere, and many women talked about feeling less pressure and being more comfortable in their own surroundings. Those who engaged in online peer support sessions described how they felt less overwhelmed about meeting new people when they could do it online rather than needing to walk into somewhere. Others really valued the privacy of learning to breastfeed and getting support in their own home and surroundings. It was comforting and they felt in control.

...and the pitfalls

Unfortunately, not all women in our research viewed online breastfeeding support so positively. Although many did agree that online support was better than having no support, many struggled with the format and practicalities. For example, many found it difficult to receive the support they needed around a painful latch, particularly if they were trying to access support using a phone. How could they hold a phone, a baby and get into a position where someone on a screen could see them? This was echoed in other research. For example women described Zoom breastfeeding support as unhelpful when practical close-up support was needed to check things like a painful latch or tongue-tie.[27]

Technology was again a huge barrier, which divided mothers. Those living in more privileged circumstances with high-speed internet, large computer screens, or a willing and supportive partner who could hold a phone or screen and position it in a useful way, did much better. Those without? Well it was clearly more challenging or game over. Some women talked about how much more stressful trying to communicate over a screen could be when recovering from a difficult birth, after a broken night's sleep or when struggling to formulate a sentence from the depths of postnatal depression. Others found it just a bit odd to whip their breast out and show it to someone over the internet!

Connectivity was a real issue. We all know how deeply frustrating a lagging internet connection, or broken sound is at the best of times, let alone when struggling with breastfeeding. In one study in Ireland many found it impossible to use technology properly as they lived in rural areas where the internet connection was poor. Some women attempted Zoom calls with private lactation consultants but struggled with internet connections. Others were simply given leaflets to read if they couldn't get online.[5]

Unfortunately, a large proportion of mothers missed out on online support as they simply didn't know it was available or how to access it. This appeared to include access to health professionals and not just additional support from breastfeeding organisations. Worryingly, it appeared that a number of women found that specialist services such as tongue-tie division shut down during lockdown. The significant pain and distress this caused women, alongside often impacting negatively on milk supply, led to them stopping breastfeeding or introducing formula top-ups.

In another UK study women talked about the fact that many appointments for feeding issues were done over the phone. One woman's baby had been put on a feeding plan as she was not gaining weight. However, when lockdown occurred the mother could no longer have her baby weighed. When she rang the GP with concerns, the GP diagnosed reflux and prescribed reflux medication, but it wasn't working. Another woman in the same study had exactly the same issue and when she voiced her concern about weight gain to the health visitor she was told to check whether her baby was growing out of his babygrows rather than given an opportunity to have her baby weighed. A mother whose baby had a cow's milk allergy and frequent vomiting talked about not being able to get a face-to-face appointment.[28]

Some women simply missed the connection and reassurance that comes from face-to-face contact. In the Irish study women talked about the reassurance of face-to-face drop-in breastfeeding groups where they could go for support, but also have their baby weighed, which helped them feel more confident that breastfeeding was going well. This all disappeared when restrictions were introduced.

It is extremely difficult to sit in companionable silence on a video call. Tea and biscuits just don't taste the same when you both bring your own. Obviously hugs or a reassuring hand or shoulder squeeze cannot be given. Empathetic body language is missed or simply impossible to recreate from one screen to another. Connections were broken, and I don't just mean due to poor wifi speed.[5]

When women could access face-to-face breastfeeding support from their health professional it wasn't the same. In the *Babies in Lockdown* report one woman talked about how her health professional sat across the room, giving her instructions on how to latch her baby on.[3] Appointments were kept to the bare minimum time needed to give instructions, with other support given over the phone. Given that we know how much women value emotional support and time from their health professional, rather than practical guidance alone, it appears that they have been missing out on much of what we know works well in enabling breastfeeding.

It wasn't just families who were struggling with all these changes to care. In some research I conducted (but have not yet published) of the experiences of breastfeeding professionals and supporters in providing care during the first lockdown, it is clear how challenging some found having to alter their care. As in the research with midwives and health visitors mentioned in previous chapters, many desperately missed being able to make face-to-face visits, or when these were allowed having to wear PPE or remain physically distant. Others struggled with seeing parents struggle, and found it distressing to try to pick up the pieces when women hadn't received the care they needed at an earlier stage. Many knew that they were not reaching as many parents as before, or were seeing fewer more vulnerable parents due to issues with technology and connectivity. Levels of stress and burnout were high, alongside increased feelings of anxiety and depression. Again, when we think about healing and moving forward from the trauma of the pandemic, those who care for new families must not be forgotten.

Thankfully, as we moved out of hard lockdowns, face-to-face support could start again, at first outside and then eventually inside. Outside support can be great... if it's not too far from home, there's a nice café, it's sunny and the toilets are open. It's not so helpful in the rain, with a newborn. Changes to arrangements were often difficult to decipher, not helped by different regulations in different areas of the UK, which led to more families missing out on support as it wasn't clear what they could access. Consistency and clarity are important when communicating public health measures and guidelines.

The wider effects of lockdown on breastfeeding experience

Practical and emotional support from health professionals and peer supporters is a really important way of enabling women to breastfeed for longer, but it is not the only thing that matters. Breastfeeding women don't exist in some sort of weird vacuum where the rest of life doesn't affect them. They can have all the professional and peer support in the world, but if their partner is unsupportive, they're juggling other responsibilities alone or struggling with their mental health, breastfeeding often feels tougher.

The pandemic and lockdown have been hard for us all in different ways. In our research we wanted to explore how mothers felt that their experiences of lockdown had affected their experience of feeding their baby. We asked whether they had experienced different issues and whether they perceived these to have had a positive or negative impact on breastfeeding.

What was notable was that two women could experience the same situation very differently. For some a factor such as having other children at home irrevocably damaged their ability to breastfeed as they felt torn in different ways and overwhelmed, while for others having their other children at home meant that the pressure of having to rush about was taken off them.

Here are some of the different aspects of lockdown that affected breastfeeding (the remaining percentages felt these had no impact). In each of these scenarios those no longer breastfeeding were more likely to experience a negative impact compared to those still breastfeeding:

- **Having older children at home: 25% positive, 30% negative**
- **Having fewer visitors after birth in hospital: 22% positive, 24% negative**
- **Having to stay at home: 18% positive, 62% negative**
- **Not having close family visit: 12% positive, 65% negative**
- **Not having other visitors: 27% positive, 54% negative**
- **Not being able to go to baby groups: 1% positive, 81% negative**
- **Not being able to go to baby clinic: 2% positive, 79% negative**

Not every parent who tried to breastfeed a baby during the pandemic had a negative experience. For some, the overall impact when they reflected on it had actually been positive. Others could identify that even though they had struggled with parts, other aspects had actually been okay. Starting with the experiences of women who felt as if lockdown had been a positive experience, it was clear that for these women, social distancing and staying home gave them more chance to rest, recuperate and bond with their baby. Again it tended to be women who were in more positive home circumstances who felt this way. But there were some elements of the restrictions that actually helped breastfeeding. For example, some mothers talked about having more time to focus on breastfeeding, particularly if they were struggling with issues such as latch. They didn't need to worry about a stream of visitors or getting out and about. Instead they had the time to focus on feeding, often sitting around the house with their top off having lots of skin-to-skin and latching practice.

The lack of visitors – particularly the unhelpful ones – was echoed in other ways. On a practical level women weren't hosting guests or being exhausted by a constant stream of company. Negative opinions, directly expressed or otherwise, were also reduced, as was unhelpful advice or pressure to parent in a certain way. Additionally, no one was asking to hold the baby and refusing to give them back even when they clearly wanted a feed. All of this time and reduced pressure led to some mothers noting that they found it much easier to breastfeed responsively, i.e. whenever their baby wanted to feed. We know that responsive feeding is linked to longer breastfeeding duration and fewer difficulties. This is because frequent, baby-led feeding helps send a signal to the body to make more milk. Trying to reduce or schedule feeds can have the opposite impact, as the body starts to reduce milk production as it thinks the milk isn't needed.

For some women, partners working from home or being furloughed meant that they were able to be more hands on, helping directly with the baby or looking after the mother while she breastfed. This made a huge difference from a both a practical and an emotional support perspective. On the subject of work, furlough and home-working also helped mothers who were about to return to work after maternity leave. A number of mothers commented that they didn't need to worry about expressing milk, introducing formula or working out how they would feed their baby, as they could stay home with their baby for longer, or have childcare that allowed them to carry on feeding. This was also reflected in research in the US[17] and Belgium,[29] where mothers felt that they had been given longer at home with their babies, allowing them to better establish and continue breastfeeding.

However, for those who found their lockdown experiences

negative, there was a direct impact on breastfeeding. For example, many mothers talked about how they felt socially and emotionally isolated from others at a time when they felt really vulnerable. Many had supportive family who they wanted to see, and they had been looking forward to having them visit. This was echoed in another study. Women missed the social and emotional connection of face-to-face support – both formal and from friends and family. Women wanted their mothers or grandmothers there with them to reassure and help them and this wasn't possible.[5]

This lack of support was often exacerbated by having other older children at home due to school and childcare closures. There was no option for someone else to take the children for a break or entertain them in other ways. Many talked about partners who worked on the frontline having to work even harder, or even be separated from the rest of the family due to fears they would pass the virus on. This meant that the burden of childcare fell solely to the mother, leaving her feeling overwhelmed and desperate to try anything that she felt might make a difference.

Of course, breastfeeding mothers can also be at work in frontline jobs themselves. Some women talked about how the intense pressures at work prevented them from expressing so regularly, so their milk supply dropped. Busy schedules, stress and lots of personal protective equipment (PPE) meant they were hot and dehydrated and had little time to express, meaning they had less milk or were feeling very engorged.

Inequities in experience

Experiences of lockdown were further affected by maternal background. Mothers with a higher level of education were more likely to feel the impact of not having visitors at home, and experience not being able to go to baby groups or baby clinic as negative, suggesting that perhaps these mothers have more positive breastfeeding encounters with those they would typically meet through these avenues, or perhaps are more likely to want to access them.

There was also a wider impact of demographic background upon lockdown experience, as you might expect. There was a lot of talk about 'we are all weathering the same storm' when it came to lockdowns, but as many people rightly pointed out, your experience of the storm was very different according to which vessel you were sailing (or clinging on to). Those who experienced lockdown in more privileged circumstances found lockdown relatively easier. That is not to say of course that they experienced no difficulties, or that other elements of their lives did not make the experience challenging. However, their living circumstances tended not to contribute to these challenges.

For example, where mothers were living in areas where they felt able to get out for regular local walks, their experience was easier. The same was true for those who had access to a private garden. A good wifi connection also made things easier. This is logical – having space, the chance to get out and about in nature and ways to connect with others removed or at least reduced some of the negative sides of lockdown. Conversely, if you were stuck in a small higher-floor flat, with little access to safe walks or space to sit outside, and your only internet connection was via an expensive data bundle on your phone, then things felt a lot tougher.

Indeed, these aspects were linked to whether a mother continued breastfeeding or not. Mothers who had access to high-speed wifi and a private garden were more likely to continue breastfeeding. Why? Because mental health and wellbeing are closely tied to continuing to breastfeed. Although mental health difficulties should not directly affect milk production, often formula is suggested as a way to make things easier. This often isn't the case. After all babies still need feeding and now bottles need to be prepared too, and the hormones produced when breastfeeding can actually help the body deal with stress from a physiological perspective.

However, when you're feeling miserable, exhausted or anxious, everything feels difficult and breastfeeding often gets blamed. Formula can feel like something you can at least try – and other people often put pressure on you to do so, suggesting that they might help feed the baby, or that bottle-feeding will help you feel more rested. Unfortunately this is often not the case and there is actually growing evidence that overall, once preparing bottles and settling babies back to sleep is taken into account, breastfeeding mothers actually get more sleep than those who formula feed.

The inequity in access to support between women from BAME and White groups was also of significant concern. In the UK women from BAME groups are more likely to initiate breastfeeding and continue for longer than women from White backgrounds.[23] However, this is not to say that they do not experience problems and need support. In our research we found that women from BAME groups were less likely to feel that they had been able to access good practical support with breastfeeding during the lockdown. One reason for this may have been the way in which support is delivered. Growing research is highlighting how women from BAME backgrounds often don't find breastfeeding support to be culturally relevant or sensitive, or that it is targeted towards and led by White communities.[30] Was that a heightened issue during the pandemic?

Opportunistic formula milk marketing

Unfortunately the breastmilk substitute industry saw the pandemic-related effects on postnatal care and women's anxieties as an opportunity to promote their products, under the guise of offering breastfeeding support. In our research we asked mothers whether they had seen any targeted adverts on social media from the formula industry, such as 'sponsored' adverts cropping up in their timelines. Of those who used social media, 80% said that they had received targeted adverts. This is despite it being against the WHO Code to directly target mothers with a baby under six months old. We asked women to click on the further information sections on the posts such as the 'Why am I seeing this advert?' on Facebook. One of the reasons given was because the account had an interest in breastfeeding. Why is this a reason for promoting formula milk?[31]

To get around the WHO Code restrictions, posts were often not directly about advertising formula milk products, but instead were adverts for breastfeeding support. For example, one baby milk company increased its social media posts during lockdown – its Facebook page published only one post in the three months before March, but then posted 11 times between April and June.[31] However, these posts (and subsequent links to videos and website) had heavy branding in the background. We know that brand recognition is a big way to sell products as consumers consciously or subconsciously recognise the branding when going on to purchase products.

Offering breastfeeding advice in this way is also a deliberate tactic to appear a 'caring' company. Research that interviewed representatives from formula companies about the tactics the formula industry use to attract customers showed that this is a well-researched approach. Companies deliberately work to build up supportive 'friendships' with new mothers, using baby clubs and telephone advice lines to reach pregnant women and new mothers without mentioning formula. They recognise that this directly or indirectly paints them in a positive light as they are 'helping', and fosters feelings of kindness and trust of the company, eventually boosting sales.

There were a number of queries and complaints about to the accuracy of some of the information shared by formula companies. Mothers who saw the adverts reported finding them worrying and affecting confidence in breastfeeding.[31] In particular one brand stated that breastfeeding women should avoid coffee and alcohol (or wait 2–3 hours to feed their baby), and be careful to eat a healthy diet to support breastmilk production. These statements are factually incorrect:

- Although coffee does enter breastmilk at a low level, research suggests that mothers need to ingest over 750mg a day for any significant impact on the infant (approximately five standard-sized cups of coffee, although caffeine is also found in tea, sports drinks and chocolate). And even then the 'impact' tends to be short-lived (increased fussiness and unsettled sleep) and fixable by stopping coffee.[32]
- Alcohol is considered safe in lower amounts. The level of alcohol in breastmilk will match the mother's *blood* alcohol level, not the level in the alcohol she consumes. For example, a 175ml glass of 11% wine is approximately two units. For an average-sized woman, that would lead to a blood alcohol level of 0.04%. Drinks that have an alcohol level of 0.05% and lower are considered alcohol free, while those between 0.5% and 1.2% are considered low alcohol. Limited research suggests that alcohol consumption can make infants slow to gain weight, but this effect is only seen with regular maternal blood levels over 300 mg/dl, which equates to around a whole bottle of wine for an average-sized woman.[33]
- Unless a diet is extremely poor, breastmilk content is not affected by the diet a mother eats. If her diet is poor, she is likely to suffer and not her baby, as her body prioritises her milk. But the wording of the website suggests a much stronger link between maternal diet and milk content, which could well increase anxiety in women.[34]

In other countries around the world, with fewer of the WHO Code provisions put into law, companies really took opportunity provided by the pandemic to promote themselves.[35] In India Danone supported a YouTube channel called 'Voice of Mums' that advised women with Covid-19 to maintain a distance of at least six feet from their infants and to stop breastfeeding until they had been free of fever for more than 72 hours, and free of other symptoms for at least seven days with two negative PCR results! This was completely against guidance from the WHO. In other countries companies stepped up donations of formula milk to communities, again despite this being against the WHO Code.

Challenges to donor human milk provision

Human milk is particularly important for sick and premature infants. When babies cannot receive human milk from their own mother, donor human milk from other mothers can be lifesaving, helping prevent infections and support health and development. Globally at least 800,000 babies are estimated to receive some donor milk annually around the world, although this is likely an underestimation.[36]

Donor milk is collected from mothers and heat-treated to destroy harmful bacteria and viruses. It is especially important that it is handled safely, as it feeds the smallest and sickest babies. Milk needs to be collected, tested for bacteria, pasteurised to kill any bacteria or viruses, frozen and then transported to where it will be used. It then needs to be safely stored, thawed and used. As you can imagine, a global pandemic with a highly transmissible virus posed threats at many stages of that process.[37] In a paper examining the potential impact of the pandemic on the donor milk 'supply chain', concerns were raised about the safe handling and transportation of milk, challenges in recruiting new donors and logistical issues with staffing if people became ill.

Another challenge, albeit a positive one, was that demand for donor milk increased considerably. The Human Milk Foundation, which is a charity working to help more families feed their babies with human milk, including directly through the Hearts Milk Bank, received approximately double the number of enquiries during the pandemic than the previous year.[36] This goes to show just how important donor milk can be for families when they cannot breastfeed,[15] and were potentially affected by restrictions on NICU visiting and subsequent breastfeeding challenges.[2]

In terms of concerns around donor milk safety, at the start of the pandemic when scare stories were flying around about the potential for human milk to contain the Covid-19 virus, tensions were high. In the 1980s milk banking suffered a considerable blow during the HIV epidemic when it was discovered that transmission of HIV could occur during breastfeeding. Fears were high about the safety of donor milk, especially for sick and premature babies – although literature at the time showed that lactation had not previously been a route of transmission for other coronaviruses, so the risks were always likely to be low. Since then research has shown that when a mother takes antiretroviral therapy the risk of her passing HIV to her baby is almost negligible if she is exclusively breastfeeding, rising to around 10% with mixed feeding, possibly because local inflammation in the gut as a result overrides the natural mechanisms that prevent the virus infecting the breastfed baby.[38]

As a consequence of this there were reports in some countries, including the UK, of hospitals temporarily stopping mothers who had tested positive from donating their milk. There were also challenges with donation due to strict lockdowns in countries such as China and Italy, which prevented mothers from leaving their homes. Others were too anxious to drop off milk at hospitals due to perceived infection risk. This also applied to potential new donors, who even if they could access the blood and screening tests needed, were sometimes too anxious to do so.[39]

However, as we have seen, there was evidence from previous similar viral outbreaks that the virus did not reach breastmilk, and soon new evidence accumulated to show that the same was true with Covid-19. On top of this, research had also shown that for previous similar viruses such as SARS, pasteurisation would kill the virus.[40] Further research then showed that when human milk was deliberately infected with the Covid-19 virus, pasteurisation killed it.[41] The World Health Organization made clear that when infants could not be breastfed they should receive human milk when possible.[42]

Steps were put in place to further reduce any risk. In March 2020, the Global Alliance of Milk Banks and Associations (GAMBA) was formed, comprising over 100 human milk banking leaders from 40 countries. As part of this work the experiences of milk banks in supporting donor milk provision through the pandemic were collated, including potential vulnerabilities and mitigations for ensuring a safe service.[43] These included:

- **Enhanced support for mothers to provide breastmilk for their own baby, reducing the need for donor milk.**
- **Increasing donor engagement to enable a wider pool of donors to be involved, reducing the risk of sickness.**
- **Additional screening for donors to include exposure, symptoms and test results. Delaying of donation until asymptomatic.**
- **Finding innovative ways to ensure new donors can be screened including focussing recruitment on mothers already in hospital.**
- **Better communication to reduce fears and misconceptions about risk.**
- **Non-contact collection and delivery processes, including appropriate use of PPE.**
- **Stringent hygiene during donor milk handling (this was already in place).**

You can find out more about donating milk and research into the topic via the Human Milk Foundation website **humanmilkfoundation.org/gamba**

PANDEMIC POSTNATAL MENTAL HEALTH

PANDEMIC POSTNATAL MENTAL HEALTH

Parental perinatal mental health is finally receiving more of the attention it deserves. As noted in the earlier chapter examining the impact of the pandemic on health visiting services, the transition to parenthood can be challenging for new parents, especially those isolated from family and struggling with the significant changes having a baby can bring.[1] Although new parenthood can be a happy and joyous time, it is unsurprising that many new parents have periods of feeling shocked, overwhelmed, anxious or low, with feelings of grief, loss and even regret at how much their lives have changed.[2] Many feel they cannot talk about these feelings openly for fear of being judged as a poor or incompetent parent.[3]

For most new parents these emotions are just part of the ever-changing chaos of new parenthood and are mild and often balanced by more positive emotions and experiences. Yet for some these emotions are much deeper and longer lasting, with significant implications for their wellbeing. Postnatal depression (PND) 'officially' affects around one in five women after birth, but it is likely that these figures are much higher. Maternal concerns around talking about how they feel or difficulty in accessing support mean that this figure is likely an underestimation. Symptoms of PND include the 'typical' depressive symptoms of feeling low and tearful, but many women with PND experience high levels of anxiety. They may also have broader symptoms including problems with appetite (eating too little or too much), sleep (again too little or too much) and feelings of guilt, worthlessness or hopelessness.[4] Concerns about being a 'good enough mother' are common.

It is not just mothers who can experience postnatal depression. Increasing research has highlighted that men can also struggle with the transition to fatherhood.[5] There is a dearth of research examining the impact of the postnatal period on the mental health of same-sex partners, but it is likely that many aspects of both maternal and paternal experiences are relevant. Estimates suggest that around one in 10 new fathers has symptoms indicative of depression,[6] although again it is likely that this is under reported – probably even more so than for women due to perceptions of stigma and masculinity in our society.[7]

Some fathers experience similar symptoms to women of postnatal depression and anxiety, although evidence suggests that men experiencing postnatal mental health issues may be more likely to experience feelings of rage and/or disconnection from those around them.[8] Fathers can experience the same challenges in adapting to new parenthood, but the pressures may be slightly different from those commonly experienced by mothers. Although there is of course huge variation in the roles new parents adopt after the birth of a baby, many men report significant pressure from feeling that they have to be 'the strong one' and look after and protect their new family both financially and emotionally.

However, it is not just men who can experience rage as a symptom of postnatal depression after birth. The topic of maternal postnatal rage is now receiving more attention too.[9] Female anger is something our society is typically not very good at handling. We almost expect (but of course do not necessarily accept) male anger, whereas female anger is very much at odds with the popular image of the 'nurturing mother'. But mothers who experience postnatal rage report feeling on edge, irritable and simply downright angry. Postnatal rage in new mothers isn't very well understood. It's thought that the hormonal fluctuations women experience may trigger it, and sleep deprivation and exhaustion can lead to feelings of irritability and stress. However, logically rage as a response to modern new motherhood makes a lot of sense. Trying to care for a small human being alone, without much support, while feeling overwhelmed and exhausted, naturally leaves us feeling irritable and angry. Anger is also a common reaction to feeling grief or loss – something many new parents talk about experiencing in relation to missing their 'old lives' and relative freedom.

Significant investments have been made in recent years to try to reduce the occurrence of postnatal mental health issues because of the recognised impacts on new families. Although research has not examined the impact of male depression on infant development, there is some evidence that at its most severe maternal depression can affect infant development and wellbeing. This is typically a consequence of significant maternal distress, leading to disengagement with their baby or not being able to recognise infant cues.[10]

However, in the majority of cases parents experiencing PND are often very engaged with their baby, most likely fuelled by their anxieties around not being a 'good enough' parent. Research with mothers experiencing depression often reveals that mothers love their babies very much, and care for and meet their needs well, but find the wider consequences of caring for their baby, such as isolation, money worries or relationship pressures, challenging. Thus, supporting mental health during the postnatal period is of primary concern because of the wellbeing of new parents themselves. Postnatal depression and anxiety can have significant negative impacts on how well parents find they can function and their wider physical health and wellbeing.[11]

A growing body of evidence now tells us what works best to support parents experiencing PND, alongside reducing the likelihood of it occurring in the first place. As we have already seen, one of the simplest things is to offer programmes of continuous support in the community. When conducted well, 'listening visits' when a health professional simply sits with, talks to, and supports a new mother, can make a big difference to maternal wellbeing. These conversations don't have to be about how a mother feels, or her baby – it is the process of just having someone to chat to and the experience of being listened to that appears to make a positive difference.[12]

Another important factor in postnatal mental health support is the development of a trusting relationship between mother and health professional (or supporter). Trust, familiarity and feeling like a relationship has developed over time encourages mothers to open up and talk about how they really feel without fear of being judged or misunderstood.[13]

The impact of the pandemic on postnatal mental health and wellbeing

Given what we know about what works to support parental mental health, it's not hard to see that the pandemic and subsequent changes to care and social connection have had a major impact on the wellbeing of many new families. We primarily need to consider two main things – the broader wellbeing of new parents, and more serious clinical manifestations of mental health issues. To some extent feeling lonely, low or worried about the pandemic and its impact when you have a new baby is 'normal', in that it is a logical reaction to the situation. That experience requires a different type of support than is needed for those experiencing more serious symptoms of anxiety and depression, which may not simply be about the pandemic and lockdown, but rather exacerbated by the effects of it.

It is important to recognise that not everyone's experience of lockdown was negative – and we potentially have a lot to learn from what did work for some families. Some parents described themselves as feeling 'happy', knowing that they could spend more time bonding and connecting with their baby and together as a family. Many women talked about the positives of their partner being around and able to spend more time helping with the baby, even if this was in between meetings.[14] Others positively enjoyed not having friends and family visit, especially if they had been unhelpful with previous babies or were overbearing.[15] Some mothers talked about being able to give their baby their full attention, feeling that their baby was more settled and happy due to fewer disruptions.[16]

However, many new mothers struggled with lockdown, even if they could also see positive aspects of the experience. In the Covid new mums study in the UK, 56% of mothers reported feeling down, 59% lonely, 62% irritable and 71% worried. Those who had a lower family income and/or money worries were significantly more likely to report poor mental health. What was fascinating about the mothers' reports in this study was that although many were feeling low and miserable, 70% felt that they were 'coping'. This shows how commonly poor mental health and an expectation that people 'just need to carry on' occurs postnatally, particularly during the pandemic.[17]

In the *Babies in Lockdown* report, the mental health and wellbeing of some new parents was clearly affected.[18] When asked 'Which three words best describe your mood over the past five days?', common responses included 'lonely', 'sad', 'anxious' and 'stressed'. Indeed, almost two-thirds of parents shared significant concerns about their mental health. One of the most frequent changes appeared to be around anxiety, with mothers talking about experiencing panic attacks and anxiety. Overall 87% felt more anxious as a result of Covid-19, with almost half feeling 'a lot more anxious' than usual. Overall, two-thirds felt that their ability to cope and parent their baby had been negatively affected by the pandemic. Notably not many parents (32%) felt confident that they would be able to get support for how they felt, either because they did not know who to contact, or because they had tried to reach out for help and found that their calls were not returned or services were not available.

In terms of more serious mental health issues, one Canadian study examined pregnant and new mothers' symptoms of depression and anxiety before and during the pandemic. They found that before the pandemic around 15% of mothers were displaying symptoms of depression and 29% significant symptoms of anxiety. This is in line with much of the previous research into maternal antenatal and postnatal mental health before the pandemic. However, when the researchers measured these factors during the pandemic a large increase in difficulties was seen: 41% were showing symptoms of depression and 72% those of anxiety.[19] Another UK study, this time with mothers with a baby aged 0–12 weeks, found similarly high levels of symptoms of depression and anxiety. Overall, 43% of postnatal women had a score indicating depression and 61% a score indicating anxiety.[20]

Many parents attributed their symptoms to feeling lonely and isolated, away from family and unable to make new friends. Relationship strains and difficulties were common, with families spending more time together in an enclosed space, with stressors increasing around jobs, health and financial security. Many family members were unable to meet the new baby, often for some time if local travel restrictions were in place, which of course had an impact and particularly affected grandparents.[15] Some mothers felt that they were missing out on many expected stages they had planned for. Baby showers, christenings and gatherings weren't allowed, and this simply wasn't the way they had imagined new motherhood. They couldn't meet up with postnatal groups or go to classes or indeed do anything that they felt was beneficial to their baby or would make coping with all the changes and sleep deprivation a little easier.[21]

The global impact of Covid-19 and lockdown also didn't help in that whole populations were affected and therefore struggling at the same time. In the *Babies in Lockdown* report one mother commented that she didn't want to reach out to family or friends to talk about how stressed she was feeling as she was very aware that everyone else was trying to deal with their own issues and worries.[18] Indeed, in one study of women in south London, participants felt that there was so much pressure on the system that they felt guilty about saying they weren't feeling okay actually and could do with some help. One woman described it as feeling like she was asking for a 'luxury product' when she needed mental health support.[22]

In another research study that interviewed pregnant and postnatal women, the change in support networks was observed to have a detrimental effect.[23] Women talked about how they would typically rely on female friends and family members to chat to and share concerns with, often having these conversations at social meet-ups. The enforced isolation broke this chain of support, but also meant that women were primarily spending time at home with (in this particular study) their male partner. Many of the women in the research raised the issue that their partner was not used to taking on this emotional support role, or at least not with the intensity that women were used to when they reached out for emotional support with the mothering role. This led to further tensions on top of the reduced support.

Some women continued to struggle with fears about infection and the perceived increased risk to their baby. In one research study, some mothers talked about how they were reluctant to go out and about or meet people in case their baby became unwell.[16] They really worried about lockdown easing because their baby would have to meet family and friends and people would expect to be able to cuddle them. Others worried about having to go back to work and the risk to their baby of placing them in childcare.

There were also broader pressures that lockdown created within family homes. Although of course there are exceptions, in general women with older children took on the role of home-schooling and caring for children and the home to a greater extent during the lockdown. Families being at home more meant that more housework was needed, which women tended to take more responsibility for.[24] Working mothers were five times more likely to have reduced their working hours than men – with the gender gap in working hours growing to 50%.[25] This exacerbated feelings of isolation and exhaustion among new mothers. They felt that they spent their days caring for others and enabling others to get on with their lives, while no one cared for them.[23]

Experience was again linked to parental background. In the *Babies in Lockdown* report, parents with lower family incomes were almost twice as likely to report feeling 'a lot more anxious' than those with the highest incomes. Younger parents also experienced the highest levels of anxiety. Women from BAME groups also experienced significantly higher levels of anxiety and stress during lockdown. We already know that postnatal mental health complications are more common amongst BAME groups in the UK,[26] in part due to a lack of tailored support services alongside the systemic issues of racism and bias discussed earlier.[27] Again, the idea that we were somehow all 'weathering the same storm' could not be further from the truth.

Another risk factor identified in the Covid new mums study was having a partner who was working in a frontline role.[23] This impacted negatively on new mothers' mental health in two main ways. First, mothers were anxious about their partner catching the virus and being unwell, and also bringing the virus home and infecting their baby. They were also more likely to feel overwhelmed, because often their partners were working longer hours, with work being more stressful or intense, particularly in health and social care roles. Complaining about your challenging day at home with a baby can feel difficult when your partner has been trying to support people who are critically ill and dying of a virus – but that doesn't make the experience of intense and lonely mothering any easier. Both are tough jobs in different ways and you can see how some families' experiences were lightyears away from those where partners were furloughed from secure, well-paid jobs.

What about fathers and partners?

Somewhat ironically, given the lack of engagement until relevantly recently about the importance of paternal mental health during the perinatal period, there is little research into how partners have been affected by the Covid-19 pandemic – and what is published focuses on fathers. Although awareness was heightened about the importance of trying to reach out to new mothers by providing online support, research shows that fathers often find it difficult to engage with programmes typically designed for mothers, feeling that they are more focussed on mothers' needs.[28] This can leave fathers feeling overlooked by health professionals.[29] Moving postnatal support to phone calls is likely to have further excluded fathers and partners from receiving postnatal support.[30]

Given that the experience of the pandemic and lockdown appeared to exacerbate a lot of common issues during the perinatal period, I would imagine that fathers and partners also experienced this intensity. We know that new dads often feel the pressure to step up and be 'the protector' of their partner and baby during this time, wanting to play the role of the traditional 'tough guy' who doesn't need support.[31] This might be increased if their partner is clearly struggling with her mental health.[32] Others felt pressure to provide for their family, sometimes putting their health at risk to find work, particularly if money issues were a worry.[33]

One study that did explore fathers' mental health during the pandemic included fathers with a child from birth to eight years old. In this sample 37% were showing symptoms of depression and 23% symptoms of anxiety. Financial insecurity and relationship difficulties were key influences on poorer mental health.[34] In another study in China, 14% of new fathers had significant symptoms of postnatal depression, again exacerbated by money worries and relationship difficulties.[35] Similarly a study that compared paternal postnatal depression rates in Finland before and during the pandemic found an increase from 11.9% to 15.4%.[36]

Further studies highlighted that for some fathers, their mental health and parenting self-efficacy was improved during the pandemic as they could spend more time getting to know their baby. Most had planned to only take a short amount of paternity leave, but furlough or working from home meant that they had more connection with their baby and were involved in more caring tasks, meaning they felt they bonded more strongly with them. For some this helped strengthen their relationship with their partner as care felt more equitable and both partners had a better understanding of what the other 'does all day'.[37]

Overall it is abundantly clear how badly new parents struggled through those early weeks and months with their new baby. Many felt forgotten, or that they couldn't say how tough they were finding things due to the constant reporting of figures of hospitalisations and deaths. But the postpartum period is such an intense time, when support and connection are vital. No wonder so many new parents are left with lasting distress and anxiety about their experiences during this time.

8

THE IMPACT OF LOCKDOWN ON INFANT HEALTH AND DEVELOPMENT

THE IMPACT OF LOCKDOWN ON INFANT HEALTH AND DEVELOPMENT

In this chapter we will consider the potential impact of the changes to care during the pandemic on baby development. This can be an emotive topic and I do not want this chapter to be a 'doom and gloom' filled piece about how we have destroyed the future for our pandemic babies. We know that overall babies are pretty resilient. Yes, they will have had less opportunity for social contacts and new experiences during lockdown, but we have a wealth of evidence that shows that as long as babies' primary needs are met, things basically turn out fine for them. At the end of the day babies need warmth, security, love and food. And parents can provide all those things, even during a pandemic. As with many aspects of the lockdown, and wellbeing during the postnatal period in general, it's the parents who worry and suffer rather than the babies. The babies are doing just fine.

I'm not just being nice to try to make everyone feel better. There's a whole body of research that has looked into what babies and children need, based on the idea not of perfect parenting, but parenting that is 'good enough'. This phrase was coined by Donald Winnicott, a paediatrician and psychoanalyst, back in 1953.[1] He spent many years watching mothers and babies and concluded that as long as a baby's main needs for food, warmth and comfort were met, most often in a loving and responsive way, then that was what mattered. Other stuff was great, but if a baby was having their main needs met, they felt secure.

So while we do need to look at the potential impacts of the pandemic on babies' health and development, it is mainly from a position of learning lessons for the future and making sure we don't make the same mistakes again. Babies have plenty of time to have new experiences and recover from the restrictions that were put on their lives. And some of the areas in which we need to catch up are more practical than others. Let's have a look.

Healthcare appointments and check-ups

We know from service provision across the whole of the NHS that many non-urgent appointments and check-ups were cancelled during the pandemic. This, as we have seen in other chapters, applied across many areas of antenatal and postnatal care. We've already examined the impact of baby development checks and feeding support being cancelled, but some mothers also found that their specialist appointments being cancelled, such as for paediatric cardiac support. This understandably left many parents feeling anxious about what might be missed or the impact of delaying treatment. Others talked about how it was impossible to get a face-to-face appointment when there were health concerns.[2]

Others were just very aware that their baby didn't really get seen by anyone other than them. Although for some mothers there was no major health concern that they needed specific advice with, they missed the reassurance of a health visitor or feeding specialist seeing their baby at baby clinic or other baby groups. Given that friends and family could not visit the baby either, mothers were aware that there was no one to get a second opinion from, or to spot something the mother wasn't aware of. In one study with women in south London a woman described how she often rang the postnatal ward, feeling like she was overreacting and needing too much support. However, during one call she mentioned that her baby sometimes went floppy, which raised concerns and an ambulance was sent.[3]

As we saw earlier, accident and emergency wards around the country saw a major drop in attendance during the first lockdown. Worryingly, this included emergency appointments for babies and children. In the first month of lockdown in the UK, the number of infants and children attending A&E dropped by 90%.[4] Some of these appointments may have usually been parents being overly cautious (or being sent there by a call handler), but it raises worrying questions about whether some children really needed to be seen but were not.

Infant vaccination rates also fell significantly, particularly during the first lockdown.[5] In May 2020 the World Health Organization raised concerns about this happening on a global scale. Vaccines were being reduced or avoided in at least 68 countries around the world, affecting up to 80 million children under the age of one. A survey of 129 countries found that 53% had moderate to severe disruptions to vaccination services from March–April 2020, including in high-risk countries such as India, Pakistan and Vietnam.[6] Rates were also down in the UK, USA and Scandinavia, particularly for infant and toddler vaccinations.

The WHO attributed the disruption to restrictions on travel, fear of the virus and healthcare professional shortages. Lockdown-related delays to the transport of vaccines globally were also highlighted by UNICEF. A study in the UK with 1,252 parents of a baby aged 0–18 months supported this observation.[7] Although 85% thought it was important to continue with the vaccination programme, barriers to attendance included confusion as to whether vaccinations were going ahead, difficulty in organising or attending and fears around catching the virus while attending a healthcare facility. Many parents said that they had appointments cancelled, or were told they could only book for the week ahead rather than in advance. Some GPs were only doing online appointments and parents perceived this as meaning that vaccine appointments were not available.

The impact of lockdown on baby behaviour

Parents were also worried about the impact of lockdown on their babies' behaviour. In the *Babies in Lockdown* report[8], one-third of parents believed that their baby's interactions with them had changed during lockdown. Parents talked about their baby becoming clingier (47%) or crying more (26%). Some parents worried that this was because their baby was picking up on their anxiety and reacting to it.

Again, those who were living in more challenging circumstances on lower family incomes were more likely to report negative changes in their babies' behaviour. For example, while just 35% of those with a household income of over £90,000 a year reported that their baby had become more clingy, 64% of those with an income of £16,000 or less found that clinginess had increased. Likewise for crying, 18% of those in the highest income bracket reported increased crying, compared to 43% in the lowest income bracket. Similar patterns were seen for parental age, with older mothers reporting fewer negative changes compared to younger mothers. However age may be closely tied to income and overall living circumstances.

It's likely that these changes are temporary, albeit obviously distressing to live through. Most people were more tense or restless than usual during lockdown and babies are experts at absorbing the emotions in the room and giving them back to you (just when you need it least). Babies also cry and grizzle to communicate when they don't have words. It doesn't mean that they are 'upset' or 'distraught' or that they'll even remember it tomorrow. It just means that they'd like a change of scenery please. Perhaps that café with the nice cake. Wouldn't we all have liked that! Let's face it, many adults probably just wanted to cry and throw things too.

Research shows that when parents feel anxious or depressed, they can rate their baby's behaviour as more challenging.[9] It's quite possible that in some cases caring for babies felt more difficult and parents had fewer coping strategies to 'just get out of the house' than usual. Many of the go-to survival tactics for caring for young babies disappeared, such as putting them in the car and driving round the block (multiple times) to help them go to sleep. Or meeting friends at soft play and letting the babies distract each other. Or popping round to family for a break (and trying to make a run for it out the back door when no one is looking). No wonder babies seemed more irritable.

Basically, caring for a baby during lockdown was tough and anyone who managed it deserves a free all-inclusive holiday in the sun (with childcare thrown in). The government has unfortunately rejected calls for extended maternity leave, but maybe they'll go for funding this instead?

Language and social development

One of the areas where concern was high was in relation to babies not having had opportunity to meet extended family or other babies, especially not in terms of being held or cared for by others. Those who were planning to return to work and use childcare for their baby were worried that separation anxiety would be increased because their baby was simply not used to being around others.[2] It's true that social contact and connection is important for babies, but babies weren't alone. They were with their parents and sometimes siblings. You don't need to socialise babies in the same way that you do puppies and anyway, they were being socialised – with their parents. Some babies might take longer to get used to being around others as a result, particularly being cared for by them alone, but these things are not irreversible. Babies do catch up, especially when given support.

Another area of concern was in relation to language development, as being at home babies were exposed to less incidental language and interactions out and about with others. In the *Babies in Lockdown* report around a third of parents were worried that their baby's language development had slowed down during lockdown, although around one in six felt that it had sped up. One reason for this was the introduction of face masks – not for babies, but for many of those around them.

Research examining the impact of face masks shows that they likely played an important role in protecting babies whose mother was infected with Covid-19. When mothers were Covid positive, transmission to babies was unlikely if mothers practised hand hygiene and wore masks. One study in Pakistan with 106 mothers who had Covid-19 at the time of birth found that just five babies went on to test positive when these measures were followed.[10] One problem is of course that proper trials in this area are unethical. We can't deliberately hold back measures that might reasonably protect infants to see what the outcome would be. We don't know what the impact would have been without them.

Likewise, in the community, although non-surgical masks were unlikely to prevent someone being infected with the virus,[11] growing evidence suggested that wearing a mask could reduce the likelihood of spreading respiratory droplets when talking, suggesting that mask-wearing reduced infection risk to others, rather than protecting the wearer.[12] However, the impact of mask-wearing on infant communication, social development and bonding has been raised as an area of concern.[13] This is particularly relevant for premature infants, who are already at increased risk of communication challenges and may spend longer in hospital care exposed only to people wearing masks.[14]

Facial expressions, including smiling, are an important part of the bonding and communication process. Countless experiments over the last decades have shown that babies are hard-wired to recognise faces and will respond to images of people or pictures of shapes designed to look like a face over other photos or images, even as newborns. Infants and older children look to their parents' facial expressions for reassurance or confirmation about how to interpret a situation.[15]

Social communication is also integral to our development and survival as a species and infant development reflects this. Babies learn to smile 'socially' – in reaction to another person – and use their own smiles to gain our attention and affection. Shared smiles in particular are an important part of the bonding process and babies smile 'differently' when smiling in response to someone else. They raise their cheekbones and eyelid muscles (known as a Duchenne smile) rather than just their mouth.[16] There is also suggestion that by watching others facial expressions, particularly smiles, babies learn to mimic adult facial expressions.[17] And perhaps most importantly, newborn babies prefer the face of their mother over that of a stranger, suggesting early recognition.[18]

Language understanding also develops rapidly in the first year, with babies making many sounds long before their first words. Watching facial and lip expressions is a core part of this, as is the concept of 'motherese' (now known as 'parentese') where parent and baby closely watch each other and mimic cooing and babbling sounds in a 'conversation'. This 'reciprocity' fuels the connection between parent and baby.[19]

The question arises as to how masks may have interfered with these important early stages of attachment and communication development.[20] One study that might offer a hint about this was conducted over 30 years ago. The researchers measured newborn babies' ability to track a face-like image. Babies were tested as soon as possible after birth. The researchers used three head-shaped images. One image had black shapes on it that made it look like a face. One had the same black shapes but jumbled up so it didn't resemble a face. The third one was blank. The researchers placed each of these images one at a time around 18–25cm from the baby's face. Once the baby looked at the shape, the researcher moved it from side to side to see if the baby would follow it by moving their eyes. The babies followed the face shape most often, followed by the jumbled up one and then the blank one.

The researchers then tested older babies. One-month-old babies would also follow the face shape more frequently. However babies of three or five months showed no preference. The researchers concluded that there may be something particularly important about the early weeks for being alert to human faces. Changes to vision, cognitive and physical development in older infants may be part of prioritising other skills as the infant grows.

Research has also shown that when mothers react with a 'still face' to their baby's attempts to communicate, their baby loses interest, appears concerned or begins to cry. This reaction is particularly strong in positively attached mother–baby dyads where the baby is used to the mother responding positively to them. The change in reaction appears to elicit a stress response in the baby.[21]

Babies also use facial expressions to work out what is being communicated. In one experiment researchers used visual (facial expressions) or auditory (spoken language) to test whether babies reacted to different emotions. When both were used together babies could recognise and respond to emotions by four months, but when just one form was used recognition did not occur until around five months (auditory) or seven months (visual). The combination of both appeared important.[22] The same effect is seen for recognising speech sounds. Babies respond much better when they have a combination of visual and auditory cues, e.g. sound and facial expressions.[23] Even young babies can recognise when a spoken word does not correspond with lip sounds,[24] and can even tell which language is being spoken (e.g. their own that they recognise versus an unrecognisable one) from a silent video of a talking face.[25]

However, although all this is interesting, what is important here is that many of these studies are based on one snapshot in time. Most studies that look at longer-term language and brain development have been based on babies growing up in significant deprivation or abusive households, rather than experiencing the relatively short-term impact of lockdowns and isolation. What is more important is that we recognise this potential impact and work on moving forward and supporting families, as it is highly unlikely that any changes that have occurred will be permanent. Indeed, while the impact of the importance of shared smiles between mother and baby (where both smile and hold each other's gaze) has been shown to be valuable for the development of attachment, it has also been shown to be very adaptable during the first year, so that it is possible to develop it if it has been lost.[26]

There has not been time to conduct much research into the impact of mask-wearing on babies. One study with older children found that children were still able to recognise emotional expressions when someone was wearing a mask, although they found it more difficult.[27] Another study with two-year-olds found that they could discriminate single words referring to an object spoken through a mask.[28] These studies are both positive, but do not fully address the concerns. For a start, the studies are of older children. They are also contained within a study in which children were (hopefully) paying attention in a controlled setting. There is also a difference between recognising words and broader language immersion. However, given that for most babies masks are only part of their lives rather than their full experience, it seems more appropriate for us to be aware of the potential implications rather than significantly anxious about long-term effects.

We must now ensure that babies are given the opportunity to be immersed in activities and situations that support their social and language development. This will require investment in staffing and expertise to reach families to catch up on any missed healthcare appointments and offer support. I hesitate to describe this as babies 'catching up', as they still experienced so much, just differently. But we must make sure we can expand the horizons of many who have known nothing but a life of lockdowns and restrictions.

9

VACCINATION CHAOS FOR PREGNANT AND BREASTFEEDING WOMEN

VACCINATION CHAOS FOR PREGNANT AND BREASTFEEDING WOMEN

The topic of vaccination against Covid-19 deserves its own chapter. Messaging around the safety and accessibility of Covid-19 vaccines is still ongoing as I write, *nine months* after the vaccination programme started in the UK. Whatever your own personal views about vaccination, I think we can all agree that the level of misinformation, mixed messaging and confusion around whether pregnant and breastfeeding mothers could or should be vaccinated is of great concern. As with all areas of healthcare, pregnant and breastfeeding mothers should be provided with accurate, sufficient and unbiased information in order to make the choice that is right for their family.

When the first Covid-19 vaccinations were being offered in the UK the initial message was that the vaccine should not be given to pregnant or breastfeeding women or women trying to conceive (although no such message was given to men that they should worry about their sperm, which always makes me wonder... if the issue was directly affecting men, would there have been such a lack of clarity?)[1]. Those first in line to be offered the vaccine at the start of the programme included health and social care professionals, many of whom were female. It simply didn't seem to occur to regulators or policymakers at the time that there could be women out working on the front line who were also pregnant, breastfeeding or expressing milk for a baby.

The seriousness of this oversight was recognised by many,

leading to sustained campaigning and awareness-raising by grassroots medical organisations passionate about supporting breastfeeding and informed decision-making for pregnant women. In the UK this included organisations and charities such as Pregnant then Screwed, the Women's Equality Party, the Human Milk Foundation, Breastfeeding for Doctors, the Hospital Infant Feeding Network and the GP Infant Feeding Network. Briefings were sent to parliamentarians, ministers, the Medicines and Healthcare Products Regulatory Agency (MHRA), and the Joint Committee on Vaccination and Immunisation (JCVI). Hospital colleagues even took the matter directly to Professor Chris Whitty (who was already very sympathetic to the issue by this point). An urgent judicial review was planned, but thankfully in late December 2020 the change was made to recommend vaccination for both pregnant and breastfeeding women.

However, although the guidelines were eventually changed, the delay caused harm. Mixed messaging, fear-mongering and a simple lack of data due to pregnant and breastfeeding women being excluded from vaccine trials mean that pregnant women in particular have some of the lowest vaccine uptake rates in the UK. In summer of 2021 very few pregnant women were double-vaccinated, with just 8% having received one vaccine (data on rates amongst those breastfeeding is less well established).[2] Moreover, a recent report from the Royal College of Obstetricians and Gynaecologists (RCOG) found that around 58% of pregnant women were not planning on having the vaccine, predominantly due to the lack of data and fears about its effects.[3] Conversely, many who do want the vaccine are *still* reporting that they are being refused vaccines or that confusion arises when they turn up at their appointment.[4]

Devastatingly, reports have emerged of unvaccinated women dying from Covid-19 during pregnancy or just after birth, because they weren't sure whether the vaccine would be safe.[5] This has been exacerbated by the changes in messaging. Many women who were heavily pregnant in the summer of 2021 would initially have been told that they were not allowed the vaccine, but then urged to have it, leaving some confused about which advice to follow. Data from Public Health England shows that 98% of pregnant women hospitalised with Covid-19 from May–August 2021 had not been vaccinated.[6] And figures from the Intensive Care National Audit and Research Centre (ICNARC) showed the highest intake of pregnant women into intensive care in England, Wales and Northern Ireland for July 2021 compared to any previous months.[7]

For context, this means that 66 pregnant women were admitted to intensive care. You could argue that this statistically represents a low proportion of pregnant women, but crucially it represents a significant increase in risk compared to women of the same age who are not pregnant. The key question to ask is how many of these admissions could have been avoided if women had received accurate and informative guidance and the opportunity to be promptly vaccinated?

Breastfeeding and the vaccine

Healthcare professionals who were breastfeeding during the pandemic faced a significant dilemma. Many were naturally worried about their exposure to Covid-19 infection. Others were facing pressure from work to be vaccinated. This led to some women worrying that they would have to stop breastfeeding prematurely in order to have the vaccine. Others considered not having the vaccine as they wanted to continue breastfeeding. And some faced the prospect of having to lie about their breastfeeding history, raising issues of probity which are generally taken very seriously by the GMC. One solution proposed at the time was that if those currently breastfeeding did not want to swap to formula they should simply delay the vaccine until they had finished breastfeeding. It clearly had not occurred to anyone that this could mean a delay of several months or even years.[8] If a mother was perhaps at the start of her fertility journey, her period of combined pregnancy and breastfeeding could last many, many years.

Of course, because this was a novel virus and then a new vaccine, we had no data directly examining the safety and efficacy of the vaccination during lactation. However, we could draw on data from other similar vaccinations. For lactation, there was typically no evidence that this vaccine would a) pass into the breastmilk, b) pass into the breastmilk in sufficient quantities, or c) if it did, affect the baby.[9] With no hard evidence that the vaccine would harm the baby, or indeed even any suggestion of a logical pathway by which this might happen, breastfeeding women were being affected yet again by an over-cautious 'there's no evidence for its safety' – as they often are (incorrectly) with many medications.[10]

However, in January 2021 the World Health Organization[11] updated its recommendations for the Pfizer vaccine, stating that it should be available for those breastfeeding under an emergency listing, which stated:

As the [Pfizer-bioNTech Covid-19] vaccine is not a live virus vaccine and the mRNA does not enter the nucleus of the cell and is degraded quickly, it is biologically and clinically unlikely to pose a risk to the breastfeeding child. On the basis of these considerations, a lactating woman who is part of a group recommended for vaccination, e.g. health workers, should be offered vaccination on an equivalent basis. WHO does not recommend discontinuing breastfeeding after vaccination.

Likewise, the UK government[12] updated the official advice to state:

There is no known risk associated with giving non-live vaccines whilst breastfeeding. The Joint Committee on Vaccination and Immunisation advises that breastfeeding women may be offered vaccination with any of the currently authorised Covid-19 vaccines.

This was supported by statements from various breastfeeding organisations, including:

The Academy of Breastfeeding Medicine:[13] *During lactation, it is unlikely that the vaccine lipid would enter the blood stream and reach breast tissue. If it does, it is even less likely that either the intact nanoparticle or mRNA transfer into milk. In the unlikely event that mRNA is present in milk, it would be expected to be digested by the child and would be unlikely to have any biological effects.*

US Infant Risk team:[14] *As for breastfeeding, little or none of these vaccine components would ever reach the milk compartment, or even be transferred into human milk. Even if they were, they would simply be digested like any other protein by the infant. It is our opinion that the present group of vaccines are probably going to be quite safe for breastfeeding mothers. The infant may even gain a small amount of maternal IgG in the breastmilk, which may even be beneficial.*

However even these clear recommendations did not stop the misinformation and women continued to be told they could not have the vaccine if they were breastfeeding. Since then, numerous studies have shown that a) the vaccine does not appear in breastmilk and b) the breastmilk of vaccinated breastfeeding women contains antibodies against Covid-19. Vaccinating a breastfeeding mother literally transfers protection to her baby. In one study of 10 healthcare workers in Israel who were breastfeeding and received both vaccine doses, evidence of Covid antibodies was seen in breastmilk 14 days after the first vaccination, climbing again after the second vaccination.[15]

Increases were seen in both spike-specific (i.e. related to the vaccine) IgG and IgA antibodies. IgG antibodies are antibodies against a specific infection or virus (or vaccine) that provide long-term protection against it. IgA antibodies are a type of antibody found in breastmilk that give protection to mucosal areas of the body such as the respiratory system and gastrointestinal tract – which is obviously great news for fighting off a respiratory virus. IgA antibodies help stop viruses and bacteria being absorbed. IgA is not produced by the body until a baby is six months old, so breastmilk is their only source of these antibodies before then. All samples were considered to have 'neutralising capacity', or in other words enough power to be able to deactivate the virus and prevent or reduce infection.

In another study, again in Israel, the breastmilk of 84 women who had received Covid-19 vaccines was tested. Covid-specific IgA antibodies increased rapidly and were significantly higher two weeks after the first vaccine. At two weeks 61.8% of samples tested positive for IgA antibodies, rising to 86.1% after four weeks (which was one week after the second vaccine). Covid-specific IgG antibodies remained low for the first three weeks but then rose rapidly, with 91.7% of samples testing positive at four weeks. By week six post-vaccine, 97% of samples had IgG antibodies and 65.7% IgA antibodies.[16] So rather than putting her baby at risk, a breastfeeding mother was actually passing protection to her baby.

Nonetheless, misinformation is persistent and hard to eradicate. We know that side-effects from any vaccine can be quite common. These are typically due to the immune response caused by the vaccine rather than the vaccine itself, so symptoms such as tiredness, fever and headaches are common for a day or two as the body ramps up its immune protection. The Covid vaccination programme has shown us how common side-effects can be among friends and family. We probably all know people who were unaffected and others who felt rough for a few days, perhaps in some cases not being able to work or look after children.

One study looked at the impact of the vaccine (mainly Pfizer and Moderna) on 4,455 breastfeeding women.[17] Overall, the researchers found that although many women had some of the typical side-effects, particularly after the second dose, in most cases this was mild. Women experienced injection site pain (72%), fatigue (64%), headache (55%), muscle pain (52%) and fever (21%). These rates of side-effects are similar to those in the general population.[18] For most people vaccine side-effects are of shorter duration than symptoms from an actual Covid-19 infection.[19]

In terms of specific impact upon breastfeeding, 1.7% of mothers stated that the vaccine had any kind of adverse impact, including on ability to breastfeed (0.6%) or ability to express milk (0.7%). The vast majority of mothers stated that there was no change in their milk production (90%), but a small proportion perceived an increase (4%) or decrease (6%) in supply. Adverse reactions were slightly more likely with the second dose – which matched the increase in side-effects experienced. No difference was seen between the Pfizer and Moderna vaccines.

There are many plausible explanations for these small effects on breastfeeding, including simply that mothers felt tired and run down after their jabs, which makes breastfeeding and childcare generally more difficult. An aching arm might affect how you hold and position your baby, or might subtly reduce how frequently you breastfeed. Fever can lead to dehydration, which might have a temporary impact on milk production. However, vaccine side-effects are typically short-lived, and should not have a longer-term impact on breastfeeding.[20]

In terms of symptoms in babies following maternal vaccine, 7.1% of mothers stated that their baby had one or more of the following symptoms after the second vaccine. However, because this was not a comparative study, and these are common symptoms that could be due to all manner of illnesses or events, the symptoms weren't necessarily due to the vaccine. There was also no association between frequency of feeding and babies' symptoms, which suggests that any reaction might be a coincidence, potentially explainable by maternal exhaustion (i.e. babies feel more challenging when you are run down and exhausted), alterations in feeding patterns due to maternal reactions, or particular sensitivity in individual babies. If symptoms were directly related to vaccine exposure, you'd expect more symptoms in babies who fed more often.

Symptoms reported included:

- **Fever: 0.9%**
- **Rash: 1.0%**
- **Diarrhoea: 1.2%**
- **Vomiting: 0.4%**
- **Slept more than usual: 3.8%**
- **Slept less than usual: 0.5%**
- **Fed more than usual: 1.0%**
- **Fed less than usual: 0.4%**
- **More fussy than usual: 3.9%**
- **Less fussy than usual: 0.1%**

Overall mothers were happy with their decision to have had the vaccine, with 89.4% strongly agreeing that they would make the same decision again and just 0.2% strongly disagreeing.

Pregnancy and the vaccine

Pregnant women are widely advised to ensure that their vaccinations are up to date to help protect themselves and their baby from preventable infections. Mothers pass some immunity to their baby through the placenta during pregnancy, specifically in terms of IgG immunity. Research into other vaccines has shown that when women receive vaccines during pregnancy, their baby receives some protection too. The only exception is for live vaccines (in which a weakened version of a virus is used to stimulate an immune response) – women are advised not to be immunised while trying to conceive or during pregnancy.[21]

The importance of protecting pregnant women from viruses is also relevant. As we saw in Chapter 1, during pregnancy changes to the immune system that are designed to prevent the body from harming or rejecting the baby mean that women can be more susceptible to catching an illness and having more severe symptoms. In addition, changes to respiratory and cardiovascular function due to the strain of growing and carrying a baby can make women additionally vulnerable. Previous outbreaks of viruses with a high mortality rate such as Middle East Respiratory Syndrome (MERS), Ebola, Zika and the common flu (which can still be deadly), pregnant women have been found to be at greater risk of severe illness and death than non-pregnant women of the same age, as well as having an increased chance of miscarriage, stillbirth and foetal harm.[22] As we also saw in Chapter 1, pregnant women who contracted Covid-19 were also at increased risk of these outcomes. Vaccinating them made sense.

In a letter to the *Lancet* written in May 2020, Professor Clare Whitehead and Dr Susan Walker highlighted how globally 131 million women give birth each year, yet historically pregnant women have been excluded from vaccine trials due to fears of infant harm, despite many of those vaccines later being shown to be safe in pregnancy, or being based on ingredients already considered safe. They feared that excluding pregnant women from trials would prevent or dissuade them from then receiving any vaccine that was subsequently licensed, putting their health at risk.[23] We know that this is exactly what happened, even though none of the vaccines contain any chemical component that is specifically contraindicated in pregnancy or breastfeeding.[24] Indeed, a rapid review of vaccines using components (e.g. adjuvants) and methods (e.g mRNA) used in the Covid vaccines found no evidence of harm in pregnancy.[25]

Balancing any risk of vaccination versus risk from Covid-19

infection is important. We know that pregnant women are at an increased risk of severe Covid infection, including being admitted to intensive care, requiring ventilation and dying from the virus or complications, compared to non-pregnant women of reproductive age. Data collected by the UK Obstetric Surveillance System (UKOSS) from March 2020–July 2021 found that over the course of the pandemic 3,371 pregnant women with Covid-19 infection were admitted to hospital, with one in five requiring ventilatory support and one in 10 admitted to ICU. Sadly 15 maternal deaths occurred.[26] We would expect approximately one million women to be pregnant during this period, meaning that although individual risk is relatively low (i.e., roughly 0.3% chance of hospitalisation), across the UK that still represents a large number of pregnant women at risk – especially when we 'opened up' as a society, increasing virus spread.

Additionally, although transmission of the virus itself to the foetus is rare, we also know that there is an increased risk of premature birth and stillbirth. Given these risks and the severity of the threat of Covid-19 circulating at higher levels than many typical viruses, the decision not to include pregnant women in trials has been called inequitable, potentially placing them at greater risk of harm than any risk of including them.[27] Indeed, figures from the UKOSS report above proved stark: during the period of the report from which vaccine data was collected (01/02/2021 to 11/07/2021), no fully vaccinated pregnant woman was admitted to hospital – or in other words, all women admitted had either received only one vaccination or not been vaccinated at all.[26.] How many admissions, complications and maternal lives would have been avoided by allowing the choice of vaccination for pregnant women? What risk had exclusion from trials created due to its probable impact upon uptake?

However, despite this exclusion, data on the impact of vaccination during pregnancy did start to emerge. Although pregnant women were not eligible for inclusion in trials, this doesn't mean that no pregnant women participated. Those in the trials were asked to avoid pregnancy, but not all pregnancies are planned. This meant we had natural data on two things: impact on pregnancy rate and the outcomes of the pregnancies. First, pregnancy rates were equal in the vaccine and control groups, suggesting that there was no impact of the vaccine on whether a woman could fall (accidentally) pregnant. Second, there was no significant difference in miscarriage rates between the groups, although the overall numbers are low. Data from studies in mice also show no impact of the vaccine on miscarriage or harm to offspring.[28]

This did not prevent numerous rumours and stories circulating on social media in particular about whether the vaccine could be harmful during pregnancy. One suggestion was that the technology used in the mRNA vaccines such as Pfizer was untested and could be harmful. This likely came about because as a general population we had not heard of this type of vaccine before (or indeed paid much attention to the fact that there are different types of vaccine or how they work). However, trials of mRNA vaccines in human participants began over 15 years ago in 2006. In addition, as the mRNA vaccines are not live, do not enter cell nuclei and are degraded and removed from the body there is no logical biological mechanism for harm in pregnancy.[29]

Another idea was that the antibodies developed in reaction to the vaccine could damage the placenta. In a review article Dr Victoria Male points out that if this were the case, the same would be true for antibodies produced in response to Covid-19 infection and we would expect to see a higher rate of miscarriage among those infected. Research suggests this is simply not the case.[30]

One area that has also been discussed is the impact of fever in reaction to the Covid-19 vaccine. Prolonged fevers, especially during the first trimester of pregnancy, can increase the risk of congenital defects in the baby. However, this needs to be considered from all angles. Firstly, the absolute risk of congenital defects due to fever alone is very low. Secondly, the evidence is typically from studies of maternal infection and illness, where fever is significant and prolonged.[31] Although side-effects from the vaccine are relatively common, an actual fever (rather than just feeling a bit warmer) is one of the less common side-effects and typically is not prolonged. A fever from catching the virus itself would likely last longer.

Notably, in one study that looked at self-reported symptoms after vaccination from the 'V-safe after vaccination health checker' surveillance system in the US, data from 35,691 pregnant women found that side-effects such as headache, myalgia, chills and fever were actually reported less frequently than by those who were not pregnant (although pregnant women were more likely to report arm pain).[32] Of those women who had a completed pregnancy due to giving birth or miscarrying (n = 827), 86.1% had a live birth, although most were vaccinated in their third trimester, which means this does not tell us much about early pregnancy risk. Those who miscarried were typically in their first trimester (92.3% of miscarriages).

There was one stillbirth, no neonatal deaths and 9.4% of babies were born prematurely. Overall 3.2% of babies were considered small for gestational age and 2.2% had major congenital anomalies. Although there are limitations to comparing these outcomes to those in the non-vaccinated population (such as who reported data and timing of vaccination excluding outcomes for those in earlier trimesters) there appear to be no differences in pregnancy outcomes for those who have been vaccinated.

These findings were replicated in another study that matched pregnant women and non-pregnant women who received two doses of the vaccine.[33] Women completed a questionnaire 1–4 weeks after the second dose and were sent a second questionnaire after their calculated due date. Fever, aches and pains and headaches were less common among the pregnant women. This might be due to a lower immune response during pregnancy to the vaccine; although all pregnant women responded to the vaccine and had Covid antibodies, these were at lower levels than in the non-pregnant group. However, the important point is that all the women produced antibodies.

In terms of pregnancy complications, again these were not significantly higher than would be naturally expected:

- **Uterine contractions: first dose 1.3%; second dose 6.4%**
- **Vaginal bleeding: first dose 0.3%; second dose 1.5%**
- **Pre-labour rupture of membranes: first dose 0.0%; second dose 0.8%**

For those who had given birth (n = 57), mean gestational age at delivery was 39.5 weeks with no premature births, no stillbirths or neonatal deaths and two babies admitted to neonatal care. Although the numbers are low to compare against expected outcomes, these data raise no concerns.

Meanwhile, in the US the American Society for Reproductive Medicine (ASRM)[34] has stated that Covid vaccination does not increase the risk of miscarriage, does not affect placental development and the vaccine itself does not cross the placenta (it remains localised in the arm for a few days before being destroyed). However, antibodies to Covid do cross the placenta and offer the baby some protection after birth. Therefore vaccination should be offered to all pregnant women.

Studies that have examined antibody transfer to the baby during pregnancy have been very positive. Initial case studies showed that Covid-specific IgG antibodies appeared to transfer to the baby after a pregnant woman is vaccinated.[35] Larger studies then replicated this. For example, in one study in the US 27 pregnant women were vaccinated against Covid-19. All but one woman developed antibodies in response. Only three babies did not test positive for antibodies, including one set of twins – but both mothers had received their first vaccine dose less than three weeks before delivery, suggesting it may take time to build a transferable response.[36]

This was also seen in another study that examined transfer of antibodies by stage of pregnancy, which found higher antibody levels in the cord blood of infants whose mother was infected or vaccinated in the second trimester compared to the third trimester. One explanation for this was that the grouping of all mothers in the third trimester together meant that mothers who had a vaccine or infection close to giving birth may not have built up a high enough antibody response before giving birth. It appeared that antibody transfer was higher when infection or vaccination occurred at least 15 days before birth. The high levels for those infected/vaccinated in the second trimester show that the transferred immunity lasts at least a few months.[37]

Desire to be vaccinated among pregnant women is not low, but many do have anxieties, most likely exacerbated by these inconsistencies in the vaccine programme and again media scaremongering. In a US study pregnant women completed a survey about their views on vaccination during their nuchal or anatomic survey scan.[38] At the time of the study the Pfizer vaccine had been given emergency use authorisation in the US. Most women surveyed had a high level of education (88% had a university degree) and a prior history of vaccination (78% had received a flu vaccine during the previous flu season, suggesting high positive vaccine attitudes). Overall 58.3% stated they would accept the Covid vaccine if offered. The most common reasons for not wanting the Covid vaccine were:

- **Concern about risk to their baby (45.8%)**
- **Worries about vaccine side-effects (17.7%)**
- **Belief that vaccines are not safe in pregnancy (16.2%)**
- **Belief that vaccine ingredients are harmful (1.8%)**
- **Belief that vaccines are not necessary to protect against Covid-19 (1.4%)**

Another study in the UK surveyed 1,181 women from August–October 2020 who were pregnant or had been pregnant since the start of the pandemic.[39] Altogether 81.2% would accept the vaccine when available, with 55.1% definite about this decision and 26.1% 'leaning towards' having it. However, only 62.1% would have it during pregnancy or have their baby vaccinated when born (69.9%). The rate of 'definite' responses dropped, with just 21.1% definite about having it in pregnancy and 27.5% definite about giving it to their baby. Women from BAME backgrounds were twice as likely to not plan to have a vaccine for themselves or their baby.

Women were asked to describe why they would decline the vaccine during pregnancy. The most common reason was perceived safety of the vaccine, including lack of safety data in pregnant women, no long-term safety data, worries about the speed of vaccine development and mistrust in vaccination and the health system more generally. The researchers then went on to interview 10 women in more detail. Reasons for not having the vaccine reflected those in the survey, but also raised the issue that children were not at increased risk from Covid-19 and therefore did not need the protection.

Finally, a global online study including 17,871 pregnant women and mothers of young children that included participants from 16 countries found an overall likely uptake rate of 52.0% in pregnant women and 69.2% intention to vaccinate children if offered.[40] Vaccine uptake likelihood was highest in India, the Philippines and Latin American countries and lowest in Russia, the United States and Australia. Again, the most common reasons for not wanting the vaccine in pregnancy were a worry about harming their baby, worries the vaccine was rushed and a lack of safety data among pregnant women.

Clearly urgent work needs to be done to demonstrate the safety of vaccines and help women and families make fully informed decisions about being vaccinated. It is completely understandable that many pregnant women have concerns. They were excluded from vaccine trials, which increased anxiety that they were being excluded because the vaccine would be harmful. Pregnant women are told they must avoid all sorts of things based on the weakest of evidence, increasing individual perceptions of harm and risk. We tell women that they shouldn't eat meats from a deli counter, yet they can have a vaccine? That they shouldn't take many over-the-counter medicines as they're not tested, and therefore not safe, but a vaccine is fine? Don't have your bath water too hot but a vaccine is fine? You can understand why there is a lot of mistrust and confusion – and why an overhaul of risk communication across pregnancy, birth and early parenting is needed.

The science suggests that the vaccines are safe for pregnant women, based on how they work, the number of women who have already been vaccinated and our knowledge from previous vaccines. But to gain women's confidence and trust it's going to take a lot more than saying 'you really should book your jab you know'. We have plenty of evidence about what works to reverse vaccine hesitancy. Increasing knowledge and trust in an empathetic and respectful way works better than forcing, judging, or mocking anyone.[41] Importantly, we must also offer protection to pregnant women (such as the option not to work in frontline roles) while they remain unprotected by the vaccine. Low uptake is not their fault – it is a consequence of a lack of inclusion and consideration in trials, mixed and chaotic messaging and media misinformation.[4]

A number of studies have shown that pregnant women from BAME groups in particular have less confidence in the vaccine. This gap in vaccination is hardly surprising given the evidence of systemic and structural racism in healthcare. Add in the historical harm that particularly occurred among Black African communities in the US in medical experiments and treatment in the past,[42] and medical distrust among BAME communities is not difficult to understand. Research has highlighted how medical distrust is not simply a lack of trust in the efficacy of something like a vaccine, but a belief that harm will be done.[43] It is also not simply directed at healthcare, but rather at the government which endorsed previous medical harms.[44] Given the increased risk of Covid-19 to those from BAME groups this is an area that needs to be prioritised to offer more individualised and sensitive support. Families need questions and concerns directly answered so that they have the information and tools to make decisions that are right for their families. More broadly, policy makers must examine how systemic racism and harm caused in previous generations continues to affect families experiences of healthcare today. These must be tackled rather than simply urging people to get vaccinated.

In summary, is it clear that miscommunication and misunderstanding of the healthcare needs of breastfeeding and pregnant women placed many at risk, or forced them to make unnecessary choices. Exacerbated by fearmongering in the media and a lack of recognition of the importance of breastfeeding for many women, it is essential now that messaging and the opportunity to be vaccinated is straightforward and inclusive. We must listen to the concerns of those who are worried about the safety or impact of vaccination and ensure that campaigns to increase vaccination rates are supportive, build trust and do not lecture or mock people's concerns.

10

MOVING FORWARD

MOVING FORWARD

To conclude, I want to focus on the future and what we can do now to mitigate the harms of the pandemic. It is abundantly clear from each of the chapters that the pandemic has affected every aspect of pregnancy, birth and early parenting, but in looking at how we move forward there are a few small 'silver linings' that we might want to hang on to as we try to support new families. Thankfully, there is widespread awareness of the need to ensure investment in the future to help new families catch up and heal after a difficult time. Much of this focuses on investment, the development of services designed to help new parents, and the need for staff to deliver care. I also want to emphasise the need to give families time and space to process what has happened, and any support they need to heal.

The *Babies in Lockdown* report[1] calls for three main areas of investment:

1. A one-off Baby Boost to enable local services to support families who have had a baby during or close to lockdown.
2. A new Parent-Infant Premium providing new funding for local commissioners, targeted at improving outcomes for the most vulnerable children.
3. Significant and sustained investment in core funding to support families from conception to age two and beyond, including in statutory services, charities and community groups.

These recommendations were echoed a year later in a report by the Petitions Committee (which considers e-petitions submitted on the UK parliament website) into the impact of Covid-19 on new parents.[2] Although the report recognises that many restrictions have now been lifted, it highlights how the disruption caused during the pandemic has and continues to have a significant impact on new parents. Specifically, it recognises that many parents are still without full access to support services, alongside challenges with access to childcare and returning to work in a difficult post-pandemic environment – all of which has had a cumulative impact on mental health. The report highlights the need for a sustained focus from the government to support new parents, specifically by:

- **Publishing a dedicated Covid-19 recovery strategy for new parents**
- **Providing additional funding and resources to allow catch-up mental health support for new parents impacted by Covid-19 and accelerate planned capacity-building in perinatal mental health services**
- **Funding local authorities in order to arrange in-person visits to new parents by the appropriate local authority, voluntary organisation, or health visiting staff by the end of the year**
- **Reviewing monitoring and enforcement activity relating to employers' health and safety obligations to pregnant women**
- **Legislating as soon as possible to introduce the planned extension of redundancy protections for new and expectant mothers**
- **Commissioning a review into the funding and affordability of childcare, to consider how to provide greater financial security to the sector following the pandemic and ensure childcare provision meets the needs of new parents seeking to return to work**

There is an emphasis in the recommendations of both reports above on ensuring that support is targeted towards the most vulnerable families. That will include those who missed out on access to online support due to poverty or digital exclusion, or for whom living circumstances during lockdowns were the most challenging. Looking at the differing experiences within the report and other research, personalised and relevant support should be adapted to those mothers who were younger, living on lower incomes and from Black, Asian and minority ethnic groups. Although many families found the changes to care during lockdown challenging (to say the least), these specific groups clearly struggled with additional difficulties. To 'build back' equitably, their needs must be recognised and support must be enhanced.

Building services back and focusing on preventative care is a key focus of the broader 'NHS reset' that is needed to recover from the effects of the pandemic on health service delivery.[3] A review of this in relation to paediatric and maternity services emphasised that although we could learn from and retain some of the measures put in place (such as effective use of telemedicine and video calls where suitable), we must also recommence the face-to-face services that people value and benefit from.

At the heart of this is respecting people's individual choices about personalised care; providing them with accurate information and respectfully supporting them to make the decisions that are right for them with relation to measures around health and the virus. It is also vital to involve people in designing and influencing the care and support that is put in place for recovery. This ties in to the previous point about making sure that any targeted care is sensitive, nuanced and relative to the needs of a community, rather than public health policymakers dictating what is needed.

There were calls to offer some additional maternity leave for those most affected by the lockdowns. Unfortunately, the government rejected this,[4] but did note that 'Combined with some of the other issues faced by pregnant women within the workplace and limitations on government guidance as to their rights... it's clear that pregnant women have been seriously impacted by the pandemic and experienced great stress and anxiety which may negatively impact their pregnancy and birth experience'. Perhaps they will take this recognition and use it to invest more fully in services to help new families recover, as recommended?

A core part of this recovery will be investing in the services and staff who can deliver additional support. Specifically, the State of the Nation health visiting report[5] identifies a need to:

- **Invest in health visiting – increasing funding and posts to reduce caseloads**
- **Strengthen leadership and development**
- **Restore and maintain staff wellbeing during the pandemic and recovery phase**

Likewise, the Health Visiting During Covid-19 report[6] recommended that:

- **Health visiting must be continued through any further waves including preventing the redeployment of health visitors**
- **A clear workforce plan be put in place to manage the backlog of missed appointments and additional need**
- **An evaluation of the use of virtual online delivery and its potential impact on handling sensitive topics and identifying vulnerability**
- **Investment and strengthening of the health visiting service**
- **A proactive plan put in place to support the wellbeing of health visitors post-pandemic**

Similar themes were echoed in a report by the Royal College of Midwives which focused on the wellbeing of midwives during

Covid-19, including consideration of what steps needed to be taken post-pandemic.[7] Among calls for further investment and staffing, emphasis was placed on:

- **Taking time to reflect and learn from experiences rather than simply returning to business as usual**
- **Learning from other countries where health professionals have maintained staff morale and coped effectively**
- **Being alert to the potential for long-term trauma and burnout and continue to monitor these for months if not years**
- **Explore and provide support for feelings of moral distress among staff at not being able to provide the care they wished, or viewing parents being harmed by regulations**
- **Collect and share stories of positive experiences, personal growth and creative solutions to help boost self-esteem and resilience**

The focus on sharing positive stories is also highlighted in a report by the Institute of Health Visiting, which focused on examples of how health professionals, charities and other organisations stepped up to provide innovative care.[8] These illustrate how many health visitors provided a 'safety net' for babies and young children during the pandemic. Examples included reaching out to vulnerable families, investing in new software and technology and collecting and delivering food bank parcels. Even when physical contact was reduced, many went the extra mile to try to maintain emotional and social connections and relationships with the families they were supporting.

Many of the key points in these plans focus on ensuring that we never again lose sight of the fact that antenatal and postnatal care (and the staff that work within them) are frontline services that need protecting. We have learned so much about what parents need during this time. On a positive note it has given us renewed evidence that all those things that studies revealed about the importance of perinatal care and what parents need and value were really true! But we shouldn't find this out by removing evidence-based care overnight ever again.

We shouldn't lose sight of the positives that have come out of the pandemic in our haste to get back to normal. Focused time at home with their baby, free from the interference of unhelpful advice and the pressure to be out and about, was invaluable for those families who had the opportunity to positively experience it. Likewise, we now know that we can use video calls to support parents in many innovative ways... again as long as they can access it. What is vital is that we work on ensuring that all parents in the future can benefit from these things, not just in emergency lockdowns but more broadly. Investing to remove the digital divide between families has never been so important.

Yet will this investment and opportunity for support emerge? The Royal College of Midwives (RCM) has yet again warned that the midwifery profession is in dire straits due to a lack of resources, inadequate staffing and widespread dissatisfaction with the role.[9] Results of a recent survey of RCM members found that 57% of respondents were considering leaving their roles in the next year. This was predominantly driven by concerns about staffing levels and dissatisfaction with the quality of care they are currently able to deliver. Midwife levels are falling at the fastest rate in 20 years, with sickness absence high due to increased levels of stress and burnout. Almost all midwives who completed the survey (92%) felt that the government did not value the work of midwives, yet it's not exactly a service we can do without. Let's hope that the government listens for once.

And indeed, if it is listening, there are some further questions to answer. During the first lockdown, the Maternity Voices Partnership (a multidisciplinary working group of women and families, commissioners, and maternity care staff) submitted evidence to the Health and Social Care Select Committee call for evidence regarding Delivering Core NHS and Care Services during the Pandemic and Beyond, asking a series of questions.[10] Many of these are still relevant, particularly given that some services are still not being fully reinstated, and amid whisperings about future lockdowns. These questions included:

1. What plans were in place prior to the pandemic to ensure the health of expectant mothers and babies was prioritised in a disaster situation?

2. To what extent is the mental and physical health of mothers and babies being compromised by measures to reduce the spread of infection? Is the potential harm of requiring healthy women to birth in obstetric units understood by Maternity Safety Champions?

3. How are the needs of the BAME population, marginalised and vulnerable groups being met, particularly around communication in different languages and plain English?

4. How can kind, personalised and safe maternity services, which maintain women's human rights in childbirth, be maintained with a reduced and stressed workforce?

5. How will the effects of the pandemic/service changes on premature birth, perinatal mortality, breastfeeding rates and the experience of maternity service users be measured?

6. How are the providers being held to account for service changes being proportionate, given that many commissioners (and indeed CQC and NHSE) are depleted by staff sickness and redeployment?

7. How can the NHS with its multiple organisations more effectively disseminate good practice and also be responsive to local circumstances?

8. What is the NHS doing to ensure the value and practice of coproduction with service users, even when time is short, is more widely understood within its own management, including within maternity teams in trusts?

This is a series of very insightful questions, that I'm sure many of us would like to know the answers to.

What if another lockdown is ever needed?

It is clear from reflecting on the research that if we are ever in the situation of needing to lock down or similar, we must learn from what has happened over the course of this pandemic. This includes:

- Communicating risk appropriately to pregnant women and new parents. We must recognise that both sides of the picture must be considered – what is the risk to a pregnant woman from the virus, and what is the risk to her if she becomes so anxious that she avoids care? Communication needs to be nuanced and contextualised to families' individual risk.
- Support needs to be put in place for those who are high risk and working in frontline positions. No pregnant woman should feel unsafe at work. For pregnant women and new parents feeling concerned about a workplace safety or rights situation, the Pregnant Then Screwed website is a wealth of information and support: pregnantthenscrewed.com/Covid-19
- Face-to-face support must continue where possible and certainly for physical issues.
- Broader promotion and awareness of what support is available locally and online.
- We must address the digital divide so that all families can access high-quality online care. It is important to recognise that many new families found great support online and we can learn from this. But we also must recognise that many less privileged families were excluded. We must hear their voices and stories and learn from their experiences.
- Build on existing tools and broaden their use to ensure all families receive support and information. A good example

is how the Best Beginnings Baby Buddy app helped support pregnant and new parents who used it through the lockdown.

- Midwives and health visitors must not be redeployed. If anything we need to draw on those with experience in related roles to further complement the workforce and enable enhanced support to be delivered.

- We must recognise the need for support and contact, especially during the early months of pregnancy. We need to balance the risk from the virus against ensuring that new parents are not isolated and alone. In the 'paediatric and maternity services reset' review a core aspect was ensuring there was a balance between recognising the harms of the virus and physical, psychological, social and economic wellbeing.

- We must ensure that pregnant and breastfeeding women have the opportunity to participate in any treatment trials, where safe, and access to medications/vaccines deemed safe and necessary. We must tackle vaccine myths and misinformation to enable more to make an informed decision on what is right for them.

- A bigger and much broader job is to continue to fight against communication in the media that is used to manipulate and mislead people. This includes cracking down on the formula milk industry's ability to circumvent that WHO Code of breastmilk substitute marketing on social media with inaccurate information.

Supporting new parents to recover and heal from their experiences

Many of the suggestions put forward are focused quite rightly on investing in the workforce and support needed to help new families 'catch up' and to ensure the backlog of care can be met. However, major emphasis should also be placed on providing support to those affected by their pregnancy, birth and postnatal care experiences so that they can talk, process and heal. As we have seen throughout the book, there has been a phenomenal rise in antenatal and postnatal depression and anxiety, alongside increased stress. I think many of us in the population as a whole are exhausted and on edge. We all need time to adjust and come to terms with what has happened.

Indeed, recognising the harms that have occurred is important in moving forward. Setting aside discussion of all the changes and regulations that were implemented to stop the virus and looking forward, it's important to acknowledge how much many pregnant women and new families have sacrificed in terms of their physical, emotional and social health and wellbeing – often when they themselves were not at high risk from the virus. To support those most affected we need to see an investment in support services for perinatal health issues including antenatal and postnatal anxiety and depression, parenting stress and breastfeeding and birth trauma caused by damaging experiences. Preventing Covid-19 infection was important, but now we need an intervention to help families heal from the damage that has come in its wake.

IF YOU'RE READING
THIS AS A NEW PARENT

If you're reading this as a new parent, please know that we see you. Please know that we understand how difficult these early months of your baby's life may have been for you. Please know that we are doing everything we can to campaign and push for enhanced support for you and your baby going forward. You haven't been forgotten, as you might so often have felt.

Many new parents I have spoken to over the last 18 months have been hesitant to talk about how all this has made them feel. You might feel like you didn't have it that bad compared to other people. Perhaps your job was secure, and you and your partner were working from home. Perhaps you weren't struggling financially. Perhaps no one you knew was vulnerable or affected physically by the virus.

But that doesn't mean it wasn't tough. So many parts of what you had imagined your pregnancy, birth and baby's first months would be like just didn't happen or happened in a very different way. I know some parents actually found the change of pace and distance from particular others a positive time, but there have been so many aspects that have left many parents feeling isolated, overwhelmed and just frankly exhausted.

Why? Well there's the obvious fact of having lived through a pandemic and everything that brings. Even if you're secure and healthy that doesn't mean you weren't worried about your job, family or health. Then there's the isolation. The limited physical horizons. The limited interactions. The repetition and mundanity of every day. It's exhausting.

Physical distancing and changed interactions with others was also challenging. When you have a new baby, one of the best (although sometimes most irritating) things is family, friends and strangers in the street stopping and cooing and congratulating you on your baby. Instead we had people staying distant, even backing away or recoiling. Absent smiles behind masks. A lack of touch, smiles and general eye contact. Fear instead of pride.

Then there was the isolation from friends and family at a time that is usually so joyful. Missing others. Worrying about them. Wondering when you would get to see and touch them face-to-face.

And all of this is before we even factor in the experience of caring for a baby during lockdown. We simply aren't meant to parent and care for small people in isolation – but that's what the pandemic forced so many new families to do. Even in the most positive circumstances, with an involved and caring partner, it's still exhausting. You might not notice it day-to-day but suddenly you wake up one day feeling wrung out. Or maybe it hits you when you start to meet up with people again and realise the difference and what you've missed.

What makes it so exhausting? Well here are just a few ideas...

A lack of social interaction can make you feel lonely and overwhelmed. Separation from family and friends means a lack of non-verbal interaction, affection and touch. Zoom is great but it's hard to just hang out and say nothing as you might face-to-face. Maybe your partner was home but was working all day, locked away in an office or bedroom. Maybe you didn't have chance to make new parent friends. Of course, there were possible Zoom postnatal meet-ups but again... it's a bit odd sat drinking tea on your own staring at small boxes on a screen compared to the companionable silence of being together watching your babies roll around on the floor. I also think the lack of reinforcement and reassurance that comes from kindly strangers left a void here. You might not think it immediately, but there's something very affirmative about a total stranger beaming in excitement into your pram or sling.

Reduced contact with others may also have made you feel more anxious about your baby's behaviour and development, especially as a first-time parent. It's so reassuring to see that a friend's new baby cries too. Or won't be put down. Or refuses to sleep during the day. When family can't visit there are fewer opportunities for them to casually say 'Oh, yes, you were just like that! It passed'. Baby groups being cancelled also removed the opportunity for you to check out small concerns casually with a group leader or health visitor.

And then there's the monotony of caring for a small person... but amplified. You love your baby very much and may love being in the parenting role. But whenever you have a baby there is a lot of mundane stuff that gets repeated. Feed, rock, change, clean, soothe... and repeat (and repeat again). Many parents break this up with trips out, by seeing friends who have a baby, going to groups... and not just another freezing walk around the block. Instead you're focusing intensely on your baby, with fewer people to add some adult interactions to that time.

There has also been less opportunity for a break for you. As above, we weren't meant to do this alone! Even if you prefer to stay with your baby, in 'normal' life others will probably hold your baby and give you a short break. But in lockdown? Much less chance for family and friends to help out with childcare or just give the baby a cuddle while you have a nap. There was no handing the baby over at the end of the day and going out for a coffee, a drink with a friend or simply spending time alone. No hands-free time when your 'always wants to be held' baby is cuddled by someone else or fascinated by the outside world long enough for you to drink a coffee while it's still hot. Even fewer car journeys meant fewer naps. And based on all of this... maybe you had added worries that you somehow had to make up for it all. To be everyone for your baby. To entertain them and keep them busy.

Finally, there is the grief at what could have been different. The changed plans. The lack of predictability, planning and things to look forward to. Feeling like you and your baby are missing out on 'firsts' and milestones. The wishing that your baby had chance to form relationships with other people or to meet other babies. Or simply wishing that you had your baby at a different time... and then feeling guilty about that.

And you wonder why you are exhausted and low? It's been tiring, intense and often felt as though it was never ending. You've been through a huge life transition without a lot of the things we know help parents massively – connection, reassurance, and support. And you've done this without the support (at least not face-to-face) of others. It's more than okay to feel like you're going to collapse in a heap. Be gentle with yourself. Recognise what you've achieved. Rest (ha, sorry). Go slowly. Talk to people who understand. Look after yourself in the way you would a good friend.

And know that we are pushing for more support as we move forward.

Finding support

If you are a new parent reading this and feel like you need some additional support to process your feelings about the pandemic and birthing and caring for your baby, or to deal with the aftermath of the impact of this time, please know that there is support out there.

Therapy can be great for addressing feelings of anxiety, depression and trauma and helping you work through what might be causing them and develop different cognitive strategies for changing your thought patterns. Remember to seek out a qualified counsellor – the BACP website has a list: www.bacp.co.uk. For specific issues:

For anxiety and depression
- **Association for Postnatal Illness (APNI) helpline on 020 7386**

0868 (10am to 2pm, Monday to Friday) or email info@apni.org **or look on** https://apni.org
- **MIND the mental health charity – infoline on 0300 123 3393 (9am to 6pm, Monday to Friday) or email** info@mind.org.uk **or look on** www.mind.org.uk
- **The Fathers reaching out website also has a lot of support for fathers experiencing mental health difficulties:** www. reachingoutpmh.co.uk

For birth trauma
- **The Birth Trauma Association web page is a wealth of information, including specific links for partners who are supporting someone with birth trauma, or who are themselves experiencing symptoms** www. birthtraumaassociation.org.uk **. They also have a social media group** – www.facebook.com/groups/TheBTA/
- **The Fathers Network also offers support to men following birth trauma** www.fathersnetwork.org.uk/ birth_trauma_and_timetotalk

For breastfeeding trauma
You can contact any of the breastfeeding organisations or a lactation consultant to seek support with feeding your baby or recovering from a difficult breastfeeding experience. They are not just there when breastfeeding is going well – in fact most of their experience is in supporting challenging circumstances. After all, no one rings them up to just tell them everything is great.

- **National Breastfeeding Helpline: 0300 100 0212**
- **Association of Breastfeeding Mothers: 0300 330 5453**
- **La Leche League: 0345 120 2918**
- **National Childbirth Trust (NCT): 0300 330 0700**
- www.lcgb.org **to find your local lactation consultant**

For relationship difficulties

- Relate provide counselling www.relate.org.uk as do private counsellors.
- Elly Taylor has a great website 'Becoming Us' with resources and courses for parents and professionals to support them in navigating the journey to becoming new parents. You can find it at www.becomingusfamily.com.

Bonding and connecting with your baby

If you feel that you are struggling to connect with your baby, or experiencing distressing memories of their birth, there are some things you can try to increase feelings of bonding and connection between you. Lots are suitable for either parent to try. The following ideas are based on an article that Dr Karleen Gribble and I wrote for *The Conversation* in 2021:[1]

- Have as much skin-to-skin contact with your baby as you can. Skin-to-skin isn't just for newborns after birth. It can help calm and soothe your baby and help to (re)establish breastfeeding. Research has shown that it can help mothers connect emotionally with their baby, 'reclaiming' them after being separated or feeling that they were 'owned' by neonatal care staff.
- You could try a bath with your baby, relaxing in bed with them or simply spending time holding them with no clothes in between you (blanket optional depending on the weather!).
- Another way to regain connection with your baby is to keep them physically close as much as possible. One way to do this, while still being able to get on with your day, is to carry them in a soft sling throughout the day. Due to the movement, the warmth of your body and being close to your heart (recreating a feeling of being back in the womb), babywearing soothes your baby. Babies who are carried regularly cry less than babies who are not, which also helps bonding and has

been shown to reduce symptoms of postnatal depression.

- Another option is to try some baby massage, either at home or at a class when they re-open. Baby massage is the gentle, rhythmic stroking of your baby, often while gently talking or singing to them. Research has shown that baby massage can help increase feelings of connection to your baby and help you recognise your baby's cues. It can also increase levels of the hormone oxytocin for both you and your baby, which helps you both feel calmer and more relaxed.

- Continuing to breastfeed can help you bond with your baby. If you stopped breastfeeding before you were ready to do so, know that it's possible to restart breastfeeding at any time in a process called 'relactation'. Some women have chosen to start breastfeeding again during the pandemic, due to wanting to give their baby the possible protection of Covid-19 antibodies through their milk from maternal infection or vaccination. A breastfeeding counsellor or lactation consultant can help you to work out if that's something you want to do, and how to do it. You can contact free helplines for support with relactation or any breastfeeding difficulties you are having.

- If you are bottle-feeding, try holding your baby close while you feed them: giving them loving eye contact will help you both to bond. Even if your baby is older and eating solid foods, eye contact while feeding is a powerful connecting tool.

- Don't be afraid to reach out and talk to others about how you feel. This might be a trusted friend, a health professional or through contacting a mother-centred counsellor or therapist. You have both been through a distressing time and may have lost many aspects of birth and baby care that were important to you.

- If you are struggling with the memories, are feeling anxious or depressed, or experiencing feelings of grief and loss, know that these are all valid emotions. Talking and working through these, whichever way works best for you, can help you process the experience and help strengthen the bond with your baby.

- Finally, be kind to yourself and your baby – and remember you have plenty of time to bond with them, and that your relationship will grow and develop as your baby does.

I'll leave you with the letter that the *Babies in Lockdown* team wrote to the chancellor a year ago. There is still time for the government to act.

Dear Chancellor,

We are writing to urge you to ensure that this week's Spending Review allocates vital funding for the youngest children.

The pandemic has resulted in worrying numbers of babies and young children being exposed to stress, trauma and adversity which, if not addressed, could have a significant impact on their wellbeing and development:

- *The Chief Inspector of Ofsted has reported that between April and October, there was a 20% rise in serious incidents of harm to babies compared to the same period last year.*
- *Recent research has shown that almost 7 in 10 (68%) parents felt the changes brought about by Covid-19 were affecting their unborn baby, baby or young child. Many families with lower incomes, from Black, Asian and minority ethnic communities and young parents were harder hit by the pandemic.*
- *When parents experience stress and trauma it can have an impact on their babies too. A range of emerging evidence suggests that the pandemic and lockdown has had a negative impact on parental mental health,*

*due to the traumatic experience of experiencing labour
and birth alone, the pressures of lockdown and a lack of
support for families.*

*The Government's response to Covid-19 has included
support for many vulnerable groups in our society, but not
the youngest. There is a narrowing window of opportunity
now to address the impact of the pandemic on the most
vulnerable young children.*

*Earlier this year Government announced £1bn new
funding for schools to close gaps in achievement caused
by Covid-19. This equates to around £112 per pupil. A Baby
Boost could provide the same amount of funding for
the babies of 2020. This would equate to £68m. It would
enable local commissioners to fund interventions such as
targeted support from health visitors, specialist services
and charities, to help babies and families recover from the
harms caused by the pandemic.*

*Alongside action as part of the Covid response, there
is a need for more substantial investment in early life.
We welcome Government's longer-term commitments to
this agenda, including the Leadsom Review, the refresh
of the Healthy Child Programme and the increase in the
value of healthy start vouchers. Decisions made about
the restructure of Public Health England must also keep
the needs of the youngest child in sharp focus. Any new
policy commitments must be supported by substantial
and sustained investment to rebuild our Health Visiting
workforce and enable effective, whole-system action to give
every baby the best start in life.*

*Babies can't wait. Therefore we urge you to take action
now to include babies in the Covid recovery, alongside
committing to longer term strategic investment in the three-
year spending review.*

Yours sincerely,
Sarah Hughes, Chief Executive, Centre for Mental Health
Jeff Banks, Director, A Better Start Southend
Neil Leitch, Chief Executive Officer, Early Years Alliance
Anna Feuchtwang, Chief Executive, National Children's Bureau
Melanie Armstrong, Chief Executive, Action for Children
Alison Baum, Chief Executive, Best Beginnings
Peter Grigg, Chief Executive, Home-Start UK
Peter Wanless, Chief Executive Officer, NPSCC
Dr Cheryll Adams CBE, Executive Director, Institute of Health Visiting
Angela McConville, Chief Executive, National Childbirth Trust
Dr Beckie Lang, Chief Executive, Parent-Infant Foundation
Mark Hodgkinson, Chief Executive, Scope
Dr Nick Waggett, Chief Executive, The Association of Child Psychotherapists

REFERENCES

INTRODUCTION

1. www.instituteforgovernment.org.uk/charts/
uk-government-coronavirus-lockdowns
2. Carr, A., Smith, J.A., Camaradou, J., & Prieto-Alhambra, D. (2021).
Growing backlog of planned surgery due to Covid-19. *BMJ* 2021;372:n339
3. www.health.org.uk/news-and-comment/charts-and-infographics/
how-is-elective-care-coping-with-the-continuing-impact-of-Covid-19
4. Office for National Statistics (2020). *Personal and economic well-being in
Great Britain.*
5. researchbriefings.files.parliament.uk/documents/POST-PN-0648/
POST-PN-0648.pdf
6. NHS Digital [online] Mental health services monthly statistics.
7. Wilson, C. & Bunn, S. (2020). *Mental health impacts of Covid-19 on NHS
staff.* Parliamentary Office of Science and Technology.
8. Clayton, C. et al (2020). *British families in lockdown.* Leeds Trinity
University.
9. Pieh, C. et al. (2021). Mental Health During Covid-19 Lockdown in the
United Kingdom. *Psychosom. Med.,* Vol 83, 328–337.
10. DHSC (2021). *The Best Start for Life: A vision for the 1001 Critical Days: The
early years healthy development review report.* London. Accessed via
https://assets.publishing.service.gov.uk/government/uploads/system/
uploads/attachment_data/file/973112/The_best_start_for_life_a_
vision_for_the_1_001_critical_days.pdf
11. World Health Organization. (2015) The Global Strategy for
Women's, Children's, and, Adolescents' Health (2016–2030).
Accessed via www.who.int/life-course/partners/global-strategy/
global-strategy-2016-2030
12. NICE (2021) Postnatal care guidance. Accessed via: https://www.nice.
org.uk/guidance/ng194/resources/postnatal-care-pdf-66142082148037
13. NHS England (2017) Maternity transformation programme. Accessed
via https://www.england.nhs.uk/mat-transformation/
14. Sandall, J., Soltani, H., Gates, S., Shennan, A., & Devane, D. (2016).
Midwife-led continuity models versus other models of care for
childbearing women. *Cochrane database of systematic reviews,* (4).
15. www.birthrights.org.uk/campaigns-research/coronavirus
16. Lalor, J., Ayers, S., Celleja Agius, J., Downe, S., Gouni, O., Hartmann, K.,
Nieuwenhuijze, M., Oosterman, M., Turner, J.D., Karlsdottir, S.I., Horsch,
A. Balancing restrictions and access to maternity care for women and
birthing partners during the Covid-19 pandemic: the psychosocial
impact of suboptimal care. *BJOG: An International Journal of Obstetrics
& Gynaecology.* 2021 Jul 16.
17. Wong, S.F., Chow, K.M., Leung, T.N., et al. Pregnancy and perinatal
outcomes of women with severe acute respiratory syndrome. *American*

Journal of Obstetrics and Gynecology 2004; 191: 292–7.

18. Martuzzi, M. The precautionary principle: in action for public health. *Occup. Environ. Med.*, 64 (9) (2007), pp.569-570

19. Riley, V., Ellis, N., Mackay, L., Taylor, J. The impact of Covid-19 restrictions on women's pregnancy and postpartum experience in England: A qualitative exploration. *Midwifery*. 2021 Jun 5.

CHAPTER 1: PREGNANCY DURING A PANDEMIC – THE IMPACT ON PHYSICAL AND MENTAL HEALTH

1. Wong, S.F., Chow, K.M., Leung, T.N., et al. Pregnancy and perinatal outcomes of women with severe acute respiratory syndrome. *American Journal of Obstetrics and Gynecology* 2004; **191**: 292–7.

2. www.rcm.org.uk/media/3800/2020-03-21-Covid19-pregnancy-guidance.pdf

3. Favre, G., Pomar, L., Musso, D., Baud, D. 2019-nCoV epidemic: what about pregnancies? *Lancet* 2020; 395: e40

4. Mullins, E., Evans, D., Viner, R.M., O'Brien, P., Morris, E. Coronavirus in pregnancy and delivery: rapid review. *Ultrasound Obstet Gynecol* 2020;55:586-92

5. Knight, M., Bunch, K., Cairns, A., Cantwell, R., Cox, P., Kenyon, S., Kotnis, R., Lucas, D.N., Lucas, S., Marshall, L., Nelson-Piercy, C., Page, L., Rodger, A., Shakespeare, J., Tuffnell, D., Kurinczuk, J.J. on behalf of MBRRACE-UK. *Saving Lives, Improving Mothers' Care Rapid Report: Learning from SARS-CoV-2-related and associated maternal deaths in the UK March – May 2020* Oxford: National Perinatal Epidemiology Unit, University of Oxford 2020.

6. Knight, M., Bunch, K., Cairns, A., Cantwell, R., Cox, P., Kenyon, S., Kotnis, R., Lucas, D.N., Lucas, S., Nelson-Piercy, C., Patel, R., Rodger, A., Shakespeare, J., Tuffnell, D., Kurinczuk, J.J. on behalf of MBRRACE-UK. *Saving Lives, Improving Mothers' Care Rapid Report 2021: Learning from SARS-CoV-2-related and associated maternal deaths in the UK June 2020-March 2021.* Oxford: National Perinatal Epidemiology Unit, University of Oxford 2021.

7. Knight, M., Bunch, K., Vousden, N., Morris, E., Simpson, N., Gale, C., O'Brien, P., Quigley, M., Brocklehurst, P., Kurinczuk, J.J. Characteristics and outcomes of pregnant women admitted to hospital with confirmed SARS-CoV-2 infection in UK: national population based cohort study. *BMJ*. 2020 Jun 8;369.

8. Allotey, J., E. Stallings, M. Bonet, et al. (2020). Clinical manifestations, risk factors, and maternal and perinatal outcomes of coronavirus disease 2019 in pregnancy: living systematic review and meta-analysis. *BMJ* 370: m3320.

9. Vousden, N., K. Bunch, E. Morris, et al. (2021). The incidence, characteristics and outcomes of pregnant women hospitalized with symptomatic and asymptomatic SARS-CoV-2 infection in the UK from March to September 2020: A national cohort study using the UK Obstetric Surveillance System (UKOSS). *PLoS One* 16(5): e0251123.

10. Moorthy, A., Sankar, T.K. Emerging public health challenge in UK:

perception and belief on increased Covid19 death among BAME health-care workers. *Journal of Public Health*. 2020 Aug 18;42(3):486-92.

11. Patel, P., Hiam, L., Sowemimo, A., Devakumar, D., McKee, M. *Ethnicity and Covid-19*.

12. Knight, M. The findings of the MBRRACE-UK confidential enquiry into maternal deaths and morbidity. *Obstetrics, Gynaecology & Reproductive Medicine*. 2019 Jan 1;29(1):21-3.

13. Chitongo, S., Pezaro, S., Fyle, J., Suthers, F., & Allan, H. (2021). Midwives' insights in relation to the common barriers in providing effective peri-natal care to women from ethnic minority groups with 'high risk'preg-nancies: A qualitative study. *Women and Birth*.

14. Wei, S.Q., Bilodeau-Bertrand, M., Liu, S., Auger, N. The impact of Covid-19 on pregnancy outcomes: a systematic review and meta-analysis. *CMAJ*. 2021 Apr 19;193(16):E540-8.

15. Chinn, J., Sedighim, S., Kirby, K.A., Hohmann, S., Hameed, A.B., Jolley, J., Nguyen, N.T. Characteristics and Outcomes of Women With Covid-19 Giving Birth at US Academic Centers During the Covid-19 Pandemic. *JAMA Network Open*. 2021 Aug 2;4(8):e2120456-.

16. Zhu, H., Wang, L., Fang, C., et al. Clinical analysis of 10 neonates born to mothers with 2019-nCoV pneumonia. *Transl Pediatr* 2020;9:51-60

17. Zeng, H., Xu, C., Fan, J., et al. Antibodies in infants born to mothers with Covid-19 pneumonia. *JAMA* 2020.

18. Ludvigsson, J.F. Systematic review of Covid-19 in children shows milder cases and a better prognosis than adults. *Acta Paediatrica*. 2020 Jun;109(6):1088-95.

19. Altman, M.R., Gavin, A.R., Eagen-Torkko, M.K., Kantrowitz-Gordon, I., Khosa, R.M., Mohammed, S.A. Where the system failed: the Covid-19 pandemic's impact on pregnancy and birth care. *Global Qualitative Nursing Research*. 2021

20. Hedermann, G., Hedley, P.L., Bækvad-Hansen, M., Hjalgrim, H., Rostgaard, K., Poorisrisak, P., Breindahl, M., Melbye, M., Hougaard, D.M., Christiansen, M., Lausten-Thomsen, U. Danish premature birth rates during the Covid-19 lockdown. *Archives of Disease in Childhood-Fetal and Neonatal Edition*. 2021 Jan 1;106(1):93-5.

21. De Curtis, M., Villani, L., Polo, A. Increase of stillbirth and decrease of late preterm infants during the Covid-19 pandemic lockdown. *Archives of Disease in Childhood-Fetal and Neonatal Edition*. 2021 Jul 1;106(4):456-.

22. Pasternak, B., Neovius, M., Söderling, J., Ahlberg, M., Norman, M., Ludvigsson, J.F., Stephansson, O. Preterm birth and stillbirth during the Covid-19 pandemic in Sweden: a nationwide cohort study. *Annals of Internal Medicine*. 2021 Jun;174(6):873-5.

23. Been, J.V., Ochoa, L.B., Bertens, L.C., Schoenmakers, S., Steegers, E.A., Reiss, I.K. Impact of Covid-19 mitigation measures on the incidence of preterm birth: a national quasi-experimental study. *The Lancet Public Health*. 2020 Nov 1;5(11):e604-11.

24. Stillbirth Collaborative Research Network Writing Group. Causes of death among stillbirths. *JAMA*. 2011 Dec 14;306(22):2459.

25. Shah, P.S., Xiang, Y.Y., Yang, J., Campitelli, M.A. Preterm birth and

stillbirth rates during the Covid-19 pandemic: a population-based cohort study. *CMAJ*. 2021 Aug 3;193(30):E1164-72.

26. Handley, S.C., Mullin, A.M., Elovitz, M.A., Gerson, K.D., Montoya-Williams, D., Lorch, S.A., Burris, H.H. Changes in preterm birth phenotypes and stillbirth at 2 Philadelphia hospitals during the SARS-CoV-2 pandemic, March-June 2020. *JAMA*. 2021 Jan 5;325(1):87-9.

27. Khalil, A., Von Dadelszen, P., Draycott, T., Ugwumadu, A., O'Brien, P., Magee, L. Change in the incidence of stillbirth and preterm delivery during the Covid-19 pandemic. *JAMA*. 2020 Aug 18;324(7):705-6.

28. Kc, A., Gurung, R., Kinney, M.V., et al. Effect of the Covid-19 pandemic response on intrapartum care, stillbirth, and neonatal mortality outcomes in Nepal: a prospective observational study. *Lancet Global Health* 2020;8:e1273-81.

29. Kumari, V., Mehta, K., Choudhary, R. Covid-19 outbreak and decreased hospitalisation of pregnant women in labour. *Lancet Global Health* 2020;8:e1116-7.

30. Bunnell, M.E., Koenigs, K.J., Roberts, D.J., Quade, B.J., Hornick, J.L., Goldfarb, I.T. Third trimester stillbirth during the first wave of the SARS-CoV-2 pandemic: Similar rates with increase in placental vasculopathic pathology. *Placenta*. 2021 Jun 1;109:72-4.

31. Ozer, E., Cagliyan, E., Yuzuguldu, R.I., Cevizci, M.C., Duman, N. Villitis of unknown etiology in the placenta of a pregnancy complicated by Covid-19. *Turk Patoloji Derg*. 2020 Sep 8.

32. Shanes, E.D., Mithal, L.B., Otero, S., Azad, H.A., Miller, E.S., Goldstein, J.A. Placental pathology in Covid-19. Version 2. *Am J Clin Pathol*. 2020;154:23-2.

33. Marques-Fernandez, L., Sharma, S., Mannu, U., Chong, H.P. Impact of Covid-19 on attendances for a 1st episode of reduced fetal movements: A retrospective observational study. *Plos one*. 2021 Jun 25;16(6):e0253796.

34. Vollmer, M., Radhakrishnan, S., Kont, M., Flaxman, S., Bhatt, S., Costelloe, C., Honeyford, C., Aylin, P., Cooke, G., Redhead, J., White, P. Report 29: The impact of the Covid-19 epidemic on all-cause attendances to emergency departments in two large London hospitals: an observational study.

35. Brown, A. *Informed is Best*. 2016. Pinter & Martin.

36. Hastings, G., Stead, M., Webb, J. Fear appeals in social marketing: Strategic and ethical reasons for concern. *Psychology & Marketing*. 2004 Nov; 21(11):961-86.

37. www.ons.gov.uk/peoplepopulationandcommunity/birthsdeathsandmarriages/deaths/bulletins/monthlymortalityanalysisenglandandwales/july2021#leading-causes-of-death

38. coronavirus.data.gov.uk/

39. www.ons.gov.uk/peoplepopulationandcommunity/birthsdeathsandmarriages/deaths/adhocs/13498averageageofdeathmedianandmeanofpersonswhosedeathwasduetoCovid19orinvolvedCovid19bysexdeathsregisteredinmarch2020tojune2021englandandwales

40. World Health Organization. *WHO recommendations on antenatal care*

for a positive pregnancy experience. World Health Organization; 2016.

41. www.nhs.uk/pregnancy/your-pregnancy-care/your-antenatal-appointments/

42. Overbeck, G., Graungaard, A.H., Rasmussen, I.S., Høgsgaard Andersen, J., Kragstrup, J., Wilson, P., Ertmann, R.K. Pregnant women's concerns and antenatal care during Covid-19 lockdown of the Danish society. *Danish Medical Journal.* 2020 Nov 20.

43. www.independent.co.uk/news/uk/home-news/coronavirus-pregnant-women-birth-baby-nhs-a9498201.html

44. Anderson, E., Brigden, A., Davies, A., Shepherd, E., Ingram, J. Pregnant women's experiences of social distancing behavioural guidelines during the Covid-19 pandemic 'lockdown'in the UK, a qualitative interview study. *BMC Public Health.* 2021 Dec;21(1):1-2.

45. Sweet, L., Bradfield, Z., Vasilevski, V., Wynter, K., Hauck, Y., Kuliukas, L., Homer, C.S., Szabo, R.A., Wilson, A.N. Becoming a mother in the 'new' social world in Australia during the first wave of the Covid-19 pandemic. *Midwifery.* 2021 Jul 1;98:102996.

46. Jardine, J., Relph, S., Magee, L.A., von Dadelszen, P., Morris, E., Ross-Davie, M., Draycott, T., Khalil, A. Maternity services in the UK during the coronavirus disease 2019 pandemic: a national survey of modifications to standard care. *BJOG: An International Journal of Obstetrics & Gynaecology.* 2021 Apr;128(5):880-9.

47. Chivers, B.R., Garad, R.M., Boyle, J.A., Skouteris, H., Teede, H.J., Harrison, C.L. Perinatal distress during Covid-19: thematic analysis of an online parenting forum. *Journal of Medical Internet Research.* 2020;22(9):e22002.

48. Shayganfard, M., Mahdavi, F., Haghighi, M., Sadeghi Bahmani, D., Brand, S. Health anxiety predicts postponing or cancelling routine medical health care appointments among women in perinatal stage during the Covid-19 lockdown. *International Journal of Environmental Research and Public Health.* 2020 Jan;17(21):8272.

49. Karavadra, B., Stockl, A., Prosser-Snelling, E., Simpson, P., Morris, E. Women's perceptions of Covid-19 and their healthcare experiences: a qualitative thematic analysis of a national survey of pregnant women in the United Kingdom. *BMC Pregnancy and Childbirth.* 2020 Dec;20(1):1-8.

50. Fumagalli, S., Ornaghi, S., Borrelli, S., Vergani, P., Nespoli, A. The experiences of childbearing women who tested positive to Covid-19 during the pandemic in northern Italy. *Women and Birth.* 2021 Jan 9.

51. Department of Health and Social Care.(2021). Coronavirus(Covid-19): advice for pregnant employees. Retrieved 24/04/2021, 2021, from www.gov.uk/government/publications/coronavirus-Covid-19-advice-for-pregnant-employees/coronavirus-Covid-19-advice-for-pregnant-employees.

52. www.docdroid.net/TupDNvL/pregnant-workers-research-pdf#page=4

53. Rhodes, A., Kheireddine, S., Smith, A.D. Experiences, Attitudes, and Needs of Users of a Pregnancy and Parenting App (Baby Buddy) During the Covid-19 Pandemic: Mixed Methods Study JMIR Mhealth Uhealth

2020;8(12):e23157

54. Chaudhry, F.B., Raza, S., Raja, K.Z., Ahmad, U. Covid 19 and BAME health care staff: Wrong place at the wrong time. Journal of Global Health. 2020 Dec;10(2).

55. www.ethnicity-facts-figures.service.gov.uk/workforce-and-business/workforce-diversity/nhs-workforce/latest

56. US Bureau of Labor Statistics, www.bls.gov

57. *Babies in Lockdown: listening to parents to build back better* (2020). Best Beginnings, Home-Start UK, and the Parent-Infant Foundation UK.

58. Ravaldi, C., Wilson, A., Ricca, V., Homer, C., Vannacci, A. Pregnant women voice their concerns and birth expectations during the Covid-19 pandemic in Italy. *Women and Birth*. 2021 Jul 1;34(4):335-43.

59. Nicoloro-Santa Barbara, J., Rosenthal, L., Auerbach, M.V., Kocis, C., Busso, C., Lobel, M. Patient-provider communication, maternal anxiety, and self-care in pregnancy. *Social Science & Medicine*. 2017 Oct 1;190:133-40.

60. Mappa, I., Distefano, F.A., Rizzo, G. Effects of coronavirus 19 pandemic on maternal anxiety during pregnancy: a prospectic observational study. *Journal of Perinatal Medicine*. 2020 Jul 1;48(6):545-50.

61. Gu, X.X., Chen, K., Yu, H., Liang, G.Y., Chen, H., and Shen, Y. (2020). How to prevent in-hospital Covid-19 infection and reassure women about the safety of pregnancy: Experience from an obstetric center in China. *J. Int. Med. Res*.48

62. Yan, H., Ding, Y., Guo, W. Mental health of pregnant and postpartum women during the coronavirus disease 2019 pandemic: a systematic review and meta-analysis. *Frontiers in Psychology*. 2020 Nov 25;11:3324.

63. Gover, V. Maternal depression, anxiety and stress during pregnancy and child outcome; what needs to be done. *Best Pract Res Clin Obstet Gynaecol* 2014;28:25–35.

64. King, L.S., Feddoes, D.E., Kirshenbaum, J.S., Humphreys, K.L., Gotlib, I.H. Pregnancy during the pandemic: The impact of Covid-19-related stress on risk for prenatal depression. *Psychological Medicine*. 2020 Dec 31:1-1.

65. Wu, Y., Zhang, C., Liu, H., Duan, C., Li, C., Fan, J., et al. (2020b). Perinatal depressive and anxiety symptoms of pregnant women during the coronavirus disease 2019 outbreak in China. *Am. J. Obstet. Gynecol*. 223:240. e241–240.e249.

66. Durankuş, F., Aksu, E. Effects of the Covid-19 pandemic on anxiety and depressive symptoms in pregnant women: a preliminary study. *J Matern Fetal Neonatal Med*. 2020;epub, 1-7

67. Lebel, C., MacKinnon, A., Bagshawe, M., et al. Elevated depression and anxiety among pregnant individuals during the Covid-19 pandemic. *PsyArXiv*. April 23, 2020. doi: 10.31234/osf.io/gdhkt

68. Matsushima, M., Horiguchi, H. The Covid-19 pandemic and mental well-being of pregnant women in Japan: need for economic and social policy interventions. *Disaster Med. Public Health Preparedness*. 2020:1–6

69. Coelho, H.F., Murray, L., Royal-Lawson, M., Cooper, P.J. Antenatal anxiety disorder as a predictor of postnatal depression: a longitudinal study. *J Affect Disord* 2011;129:348–53.

70. Brunton, P.J. Effects of maternal exposure to social stress during pregnancy: consequences for mother and offspring. *Reproduction* 2013;146:175–89.

71. Dunkel Schetter, C. (2011). Psychological science on pregnancy: Stress processes, biopsychosocial models, and emerging research issues. *Annual Review of Psychology, 62,* 531–558.

CHAPTER 2: HOW DID THE PANDEMIC AFFECT CARE DURING BIRTH?

1. Tunçalp, Ö., Pena-Rosas, J.P., Lawrie, T., Bucagu, M., Oladapo, O.T., Portela, A., Metin Gülmezoglu, A. WHO recommendations on antenatal care for a positive pregnancy experience—going beyond survival. *BJOG: An International Journal of Obstetrics & Gynaecology.* 2017 May;124(6):860-2.

2. Downe, S., Finlayson, K., Oladapo, O., Bonet, M., Gülmezoglu, A.M. What matters to women during childbirth: a systematic qualitative review. *PloS one.* 2018 Apr 17;13(4):e0194906.

3. Voellmin, A., Entringer, S., Moog, N., Wadhwa, P.D., Buss, C. Maternal positive affect over the course of pregnancy is associated with the length of gestation and reduced risk of preterm delivery. *Journal of Psychosomatic research.* 2013 Oct 1;75(4):336-40.

4. Berg, M., Ólafsdóttir, Ó.A., Lundgren, I. A midwifery model of woman-centred childbirth care—In Swedish and Icelandic settings. *Sexual & Reproductive Healthcare.* 2012 Jun 1;3(2):79-87.

5. Hodnett, E.D., Fredericks, S. Support during pregnancy for women at increased risk of low birthweight babies. *Cochrane database of systematic reviews.* 2003(3).

6. Bohren, M.A., Hofmeyr, G.J., Sakala, C., Fukuzawa, R.K., Cuthbert, A. Continuous support for women during childbirth. *Cochrane Database of Systematic Reviews* 2017

7. Maputle, M.S., Hiss, D. Woman-centred care in childbirth: A concept analysis (Part 1). *Curationis.* 2013 Jan 1;36(1):1-8.

8. Hunter, A., Devane, D., Houghton, C., Grealish, A., Tully, A., Smith, V. Woman-centred care during pregnancy and birth in Ireland: thematic analysis of women's and clinicians' experiences. *BMC Pregnancy and Childbirth.* 2017 Dec;17(1):1-1.

9. Boyle, S., Thomas, H., Brooks, F. Women□s views on partnership working with midwives during pregnancy and childbirth. *Midwifery.* 2016 Jan 1;32:21-9.

10. Renfrew, M.J., McFadden, A., Bastos, M.H., Campbell, J., Channon, A.A., Cheung, N.F., Silva, D.R., Downe, S., Kennedy, H.P., Malata, A., McCormick, F. Midwifery and quality care: findings from a new evidence-informed framework for maternal and newborn care. *The Lancet.* 2014 Sep 20;384(9948):1129-45.

11. Cook, K., Loomis, C. The impact of choice and control on women's childbirth experiences. *The Journal of Perinatal Education.* 2012 Jan 1;21(3):158-68.

12. Hauck, Y., Fenwick, J., Downie, J., Butt, J. The influence of childbirth expectations on Western Australian women's perceptions of their birth

experience. *Midwifery.* 2007 Sep 1;23(3):235-47.

13. Dugas, M., Shorten, A., Dubé, E., Wassef, M., Bujold, E., Chaillet, N. Decision aid tools to support women's decision making in pregnancy and birth: a systematic review and meta-analysis. *Social science & medicine.* 2012 Jun 1;74(12):1968-78.

14. Divall, B., Spiby, H., Nolan, M., Slade, P. Plans, preferences or going with the flow: An online exploration of women's views and experiences of birth plans. *Midwifery.* 2017 Nov 1;54:29-34.

15. National Maternity Review (2016) *Better Births.* Accessed via: www.england.nhs.uk/ourwork/futurenhs/mat-review

16. NHS England (2017) *Maternity transformation programme.* Accessed via www.england.nhs.uk/mat-transformation

17. Henshall, C., Taylor, B., Kenyon, S. A systematic review to examine the evidence regarding discussions by midwives, with women, around their options for where to give birth. *BMC Pregnancy and Childbirth.* 2016 Dec;16(1):1-3.

18. Jardine, J., Relph, S., Magee, L.A., von Dadelszen, P., Morris, E., Ross-Davie, M., Draycott, T., Khalil, A. Maternity services in the UK during the coronavirus disease 2019 pandemic: a national survey of modifications to standard care. *BJOG: An International Journal of Obstetrics & Gynaecology.* 2021 Apr; 128(5):880-9.

19. Silverio, S.A., De Backer, K., Easter, A., von Dadelszen, P., Magee, L.A., Sandall, J. Women's experiences of maternity service reconfiguration during the Covid-19 pandemic: A qualitative investigation. *Midwifery.* 2021 Aug 5:103116.

20. Sweet, L., Bradfield, Z., Vasilevski, V., Wynter, K., Hauck, Y., Kuliukas, L., Homer, C.S., Szabo, R.A., Wilson, A.N. Becoming a mother in the 'new' social world in Australia during the first wave of the Covid-19 pandemic. *Midwifery.* 2021 Jul 1;98:102996.

21. Knight, M., Bunch, K., Vousden, N., Morris, E., Simpson, N., Gale, C., O'Brien, P., Quigley, M., Brocklehurst, P., Kurinczuk, J.J. Characteristics and outcomes of pregnant women admitted to hospital with confirmed SARS-CoV-2 infection in UK: national population based cohort study. *BMJ.* 2020 Jun 8;369.

22. Panda, S., O'Malley, D., Barry, P., Vallejo, N., Smith, V. Women's views and experiences of maternity care during Covid-19 in Ireland: A qualitative descriptive study. *Midwifery.* 2021 Dec 1;103:103092.

23. Chivers, B.R., Garad, R.M., Boyle, J.A., Skouteris, H., Teede, H.J., Harrison, C.L. Perinatal distress during Covid-19: thematic analysis of an online parenting forum. *Journal of Medical Internet Research.* 2020;22(9):e22002.

24. Altman, M.R., Gavin, A.R., Eagen-Torkko, M.K., Kantrowitz-Gordon, I., Khosa, R.M., Mohammed, S.A. Where the system failed: the Covid-19 pandemic's impact on pregnancy and birth care. *Global Qualitative Nursing Research.* 2021

25. Mariño-Narvaez, C., Puertas-Gonzalez, J.A., Romero-Gonzalez, B., Peralta-Ramirez, M.I. Giving birth during the Covid-19 pandemic: The impact on birth satisfaction and postpartum depression. *International*

Journal of Gynecology & Obstetrics. 2021 Apr;153(1):83-8.

26. Romano, A.M., Lothian, J.A. Promoting, protecting, and supporting normal birth: A look at the evidence. *Journal of Obstetric, Gynecologic & Neonatal Nursing.* 2008 Jan 1;37(1):94-105.

27. Bhatia, K., Columb, M., Bewlay, A., Eccles, J., Hulgur, M., Jayan, N., Lie, J., Verma, D., Parikh, R. The effect of Covid-19 on general anaesthesia rates for caesarean section. A cross-sectional analysis of six hospitals in the north-west of England. *Anaesthesia.* 2021 Mar;76(3):312-9.

28. McDonnell, S., McNamee, E., Lindow, S.W., O'Connell, M.P. The impact of the Covid-19 pandemic on maternity services: A review of maternal and neonatal outcomes before, during and after the pandemic. *European Journal of Obstetrics & Gynecology and Reproductive Biology.* 2020 Oct 12.

29. Inversetti, A., Fumagalli, S., Nespoli, A., Antolini, L., Mussi, S., Ferrari, D., Locatelli, A. Childbirth experience and practice changing during Covid-19 pandemic: A cross-sectional study. *Nursing Open.* 2021 May 18.

30. Speyer, L.G., Marryat, L., Auyeung, B. Effects of Covid-19 Public Health Safety Measures on Births in Scotland between March and May 2020.

31. Mayopoulos, G.A., Ein-Dor, T., Dishy, G.A., Nandru, R., Chan, S.J., Hanley, L.E., Kaimal, A.J., Dekel, S. Covid-19 is associated with traumatic childbirth and subsequent mother-infant bonding problems. *Journal of Affective Disorders.* 2021 Mar 1;282:122-5.

32. Baptie, G., Andrade, J., Bacon, A.M., Norman, A. Birth trauma: the mediating effects of perceived support. *British Journal of Midwifery.* 2020 Oct 2;28(10):724-30.

33. Rhodes, A., Kheireddine, S., Smith, A.D. Experiences, Attitudes, and Needs of Users of a Pregnancy and Parenting App (Baby Buddy) During the Covid-19 Pandemic: Mixed Methods Study *JMIR Mhealth Uhealth* 2020;8(12):e23157

34. Wilmore, M., Rodger, D., Humphreys, S., Clifton, V.L., Dalton, J., Flabouris, M., Skuse, A. How midwives tailor health information used in antenatal care. *Midwifery.* 2015 Jan 1;31(1):74-9.

35. Raine, R., Cartwright, M., Richens, Y., Mahamed, Z., Smith, D. A qualitative study of women's experiences of communication in antenatal care: identifying areas for action. *Maternal and Child Health Journal.* 2010 Jul;14(4):590-9.

36. Karavadra, B., Stockl, A., Prosser-Snelling, E., Simpson, P., & Morris, E. (2020). Women's perceptions of Covid-19 and their healthcare experiences: a qualitative thematic analysis of a national survey of pregnant women in the United Kingdom. *BMC Pregnancy and Childbirth*, 20(1), 1-8.

37. *Babies in Lockdown: listening to parents to build back better* (2020). Best Beginnings, Home-Start UK, and the Parent-Infant Foundation UK.

38. Wilson, A.N., Sweet, L., Vasilevski, V., Hauck, Y., Wynter, K., Kuliukas, L., Szabo, R.A., Homer, C.S., Bradfield, Z. Australian women's experiences of receiving maternity care during the Covid-19 pandemic: A cross-sectional national survey. *Birth.* 2021 Jun 27.

39. Einion-Waller, A., Regan M. 'Knowing That I Had a Choice Empowered

Me': Preparing for and Experiencing Birth during a Pandemic. *Mothers, Mothering, and Covid-19: Dispatches from the Pandemic.* 2021 Feb 28.

40. Chatwin, J., Butler, D., Jones, J., James, L., Choucri, L., McCarthy, R. Experiences of pregnant mothers using a social media based antenatal support service during the Covid-19 lockdown in the UK: findings from a user survey. *BMJ Open.* 2021 Jan 1;11(1):e040649.

41. pregnantthenscrewed.com/but-not-maternity

42. Coulter, A., Richards, T. Care during Covid-19 must be humane and person centred. *BMJ* 2020; 370

43. Sanders, J., Blaylock, R. 'Anxious and traumatised': users' experiences of maternity care in the UK during the Covid-19 pandemic. *Midwifery.* 2021 Jun 18:103069.

44. Cheng, E.R., Rifas-Shiman, S.L., Perkins, M.E., Rich-Edwards, J.W., Gillman, M.W., Wright, R., Taveras, E.M. The influence of antenatal partner support on pregnancy outcomes. *Journal of Women's Health.* 2016 Jul 1;25(7):672-9.

45. Bohren, M.A., Berger, B.O., Munthe-Kaas, H., Tunçalp, Ö. Perceptions and experiences of labour companionship: a qualitative evidence synthesis. *Cochrane Database of Systematic Reviews.* 2019(3).

46. Horsch, A., Lalor, J., Downe, S. Moral and mental health challenges faced by maternity staff during the Covid-19 pandemic. *Psychological Trauma: Theory, Research, Practice, and Policy.* 2020 Aug;12(S1):S141.

47. Plantin, L., Olykoya, A., Ny, P. Positive health outcomes of fathers' involvment in pregnancy and childbirth paternal support: a scope study literature review. *Fathering: A Journal of Theory, Research, and Practice about Men as Fathers.* 2011;9(1):87-102.

48. Shorey, S., He, H.G., Morelius, E. Skin-to-skin contact by fathers and the impact on infant and paternal outcomes: an integrative review. *Midwifery.* 2016 Sep 1;40:207-17.

49. Longworth, H.L., Kingdon, C.K. Fathers in the birth room: What are they expecting and experiencing? A phenomenological study. *Midwifery.* 2011 Oct 1;27(5):588-94.

50. Vasilevski, V., Sweet, L., Bradfield, Z., Wilson, A.N., Hauck, Y., Kuliukas, L., Homer, C.S., Szabo, R.A., Wynter, K. Receiving maternity care during the Covid-19 pandemic: Experiences of women's partners and support persons. *Women and Birth.* 2021 Apr 27.

51. Gruber, K.J., Cupito, S.H., Dobson, C.F. Impact of doulas on healthy birth outcomes. *J Perinat Educ* 2013;22(1):49–58.

52. McGrath, S.K., Kennell, J.H. A Randomized Controlled Trial of Continuous Labor Support for Middle-Class Couples: Effect on Cesarean Delivery Rates. *Birth.* 2008;35(2):92–97

53. Kozhimannil, K.B., Vogelsang, C.A., Hardeman, R.R., Prasad, S. Disrupting the pathways of social determinants of health: doula support during pregnancy and childbirth. *The Journal of the American Board of Family Medicine.* 2016 May 1;29(3):308-17.

54. Thomas, M.P., Ammann, G., Brazier, E., Noyes, P., and Maybank, A. (2017). Doula services within a healthy start program: increasing access for an underserved population. *Matern. Child Health J.* 21 (S1), S59–S64.

55. Darwin, Z., Green, J., McLeish, J., Willmot, H., Spiby, H. Evaluation of trained volunteer doula services for disadvantaged women in five areas in E ngland: women's experiences. *Health & Social Care in the Community.* 2017 Mar;25(2):466-77.

56. Searcy, J.J., Castañeda, A.N. On the Outside Looking In: A Global Doula Response to Covid-19. *Frontiers in Sociology.* 2021 Feb 19;6:26.

57. Adams, C. Pregnancy and birth in the United States during the Covid-19 pandemic: The views of doulas. *Birth.* 2021 Jul 23.

58. Romanis, E.C., Nelson, A. Homebirthing in the United Kingdom during Covid-19. *Medical Law International.* 2020 Sep;20(3):183-200.

59. Davies, R., Davis, D., Pearce, M., Wong, N. The effect of waterbirth on neonatal mortality and morbidity: a systematic review and meta-analysis. *JBI Evidence Synthesis.* 2015 Oct 1;13(10):180-231.

60. Dahlen, H.G., Dowling, H., Tracy, M., Schmied, V., Tracy, S. Maternal and perinatal outcomes amongst low risk women giving birth in water compared to six birth positions on land. A descriptive cross sectional study in a birth centre over 12 years. *Midwifery.* 2013 Jul 1;29(7):759-64.

61. Clews, C., Church, S., Ekberg, M. Women and waterbirth: A systematic meta-synthesis of qualitative studies. *Women and Birth.* 2020 Nov 1;33(6):566-73.

62. Atmuri, K., Sarkar, M., Obudu, E., Kumar, A. Perspectives of pregnant women during the Covid-19 pandemic: A qualitative study. *Women and Birth.* 2021 Mar 15.

63. van Manen, E.L., Hollander, M., Feijen-de Jong, E., de Jonge, A., Verhoeven, C., Gitsels, J. Experiences of Dutch maternity care professionals during the first wave of Covid-19 in a community based maternity care system. *PloS one.* 2021 Jun 17;16(6):e0252735.

64. Vazquez-Vazquez, A., Dib, S., Rougeaux, E., Wells, J.C., Fewtrell, M.S. The impact of the Covid-19 lockdown on the experiences and feeding practices of new mothers in the UK: Preliminary data from the Covid-19 New Mum Study. *Appetite.* 2021 Jan 1;156:104985.

65. Bradfield, Z., Hauck, Y., Homer, C.S., Sweet, L., Wilson, A.N., Szabo, R.A., Wynter, K., Vasilevski, V., Kuliukas, L. Midwives' experiences of providing maternity care during the Covid-19 pandemic in Australia. *Women and Birth.* 2021 Mar 15.

66. Royal College of Obstetricians & Gynaecologists. Coronavirus (Covid-19) Infection in Pregnancy, 2020. www.rcog.org.uk/en/guidelines-research-services/guidelines/coronavirus-pregnancy.

67. Frankham, L., Thorsteinsson, E.B., Bartik, W.J. Antenatal Depression and the Impact of Covid-19 Mitigation Efforts in Australia. doi.org/10.31234/osf.io/ahn6x

68. https://www.theguardian.com/world/2020/mar/27/nhs-trusts-suspending-home-births-coronavirus

69. Descieux, K., Kavasseri, K., Scott, K., Parlier, A.B. Why women choose home birth: a narrative review. *MAHEC Online Journal of Research.* 2017;3(2):1-0.

70. Scarf, V.L., Rossiter, C., Vedam, S., Dahlen, H.G., Ellwood, D., Forster, D., Foureur, M.J., McLachlan, H., Oats, J., Sibbritt, D., Thornton, C. Maternal

and perinatal outcomes by planned place of birth among women with low-risk pregnancies in high-income countries: a systematic review and meta-analysis. *Midwifery*. 2018 Jul 1;62:240-55.

71. Geerts, C.C., van Dillen, J., Klomp, T., Lagro-Janssen, A.L., de Jonge, A. Satisfaction with caregivers during labour among low risk women in the Netherlands: the association with planned place of birth and transfer of care during labour. *BMC Pregnancy and Childbirth*. 2017 Dec;17(1):1-0.

72. Daviss, B.A., Anderson, D.A., Johnson, K.C. Pivoting to Childbirth at Home or in Freestanding Birth Centers in the US During Covid-19: Safety, Economics and Logistics. *Frontiers in Sociology*. 2021 Mar 26;6:24.

73. Homer, C.S., Davies-Tuck, M., Dahlen, H.G, Scarf, V.L. The impact of planning for Covid-19 on private practising midwives in Australia. *Women and Birth*. 2021 Feb 1;34(1):e32-7.

74. Daviss, B.A., Roberts, T., Leblanc, C., Champet, I., Betchi, B., Ashawasegai, A., Gamez, L. When the Masks Come Off in Canada and Guatemala: Will the Realities of Racism and Marginalization of Midwives Finally Be Addressed?. *Frontiers in Sociology*. 2021:81.

75. Wilson, A.N., Sweet, L., Vasilevski, V., Hauck, Y., Wynter, K., Kuliukas, L., Szabo, R.A., Homer, C.S., Bradfield, Z. Australian women's experiences of receiving maternity care during the Covid-19 pandemic: A cross-sectional national survey. *Birth*. 2021 Jun 27.

76. theconversation.com/during-Covid-19-women-are-opting-for-freebirthing-if-homebirths-arent-available-and-thats-a-worry-142261

77. Gildner, T.E., Thayer, Z.M. Birth plan alterations among American women in response to Covid-19. *Health Expectations: An International Journal of Public Participation in Health Care and Health Policy*. 2020 Aug;23(4):969.

78. Moyer, C.A., Compton, S.D., Kaselitz, E., Muzik, M. Pregnancy-related anxiety during Covid-19: a nationwide survey of 2740 pregnant women. *Archives of Women's Mental Health*. 2020 Dec;23(6):757-65.

79. Jackson, M., Dahlen, H., and Schmeid, V. Birthing outside the system: Perspectives of risk amongst Australian women who have high risk homebirths. *Midwifery*. (2012) 28:561-7. doi: 10.1016/j.midw.2011.11.002

80. www.theguardian.com/lifeandstyle/2020/dec/05/women-give-birth-alone-the-rise-of-freebirthing

81. Greenfield, M., Payne-Gifford, S., McKenzie, G. Between a rock and a hard place: Considering 'freebirth' during Covid-19. *Frontiers in Global Women's Health*. 2021 Feb 18;2:5.

82. Brown, A., Shenker, N. Experiences of breastfeeding during Covid-19: Lessons for future practical and emotional support. *Maternal & Child Nutrition*. 2021 Jan;17(1):e13088.

83. Fumagalli, S., Ornaghi, S., Borrelli, S., Vergani, P., Nespoli, A. The experiences of childbearing women who tested positive to Covid-19 during the pandemic in northern Italy. *Women and Birth*. 2021 Jan 9.

84. González-Timoneda, A., Hernández, V.H., Moya, S.P., Blazquez, R.A. Experiences and attitudes of midwives during the birth of a pregnant woman with Covid-19 infection: A qualitative study. *Women and Birth*.

2020 Dec 9.

85. 85. Hunter, B., Fenwick, J., Sidebotham, M., Henley, J. Midwives in the United Kingdom: Levels of burnout, depression, anxiety and stress and associated predictors. Midwifery. 2019 Dec 1;79:102526.

86. www.rcm.org.uk/news-views/rcm-opinion/2019/ england-short-of-almost-2-500-midwives-new-birth-figures-confirm

87. Hunter, B., Renfrew, M.J., Downe, S., Cheyne, H., Dykes, F., Lavender, T., Page, L., Sandall, J., Spiby, H. Supporting the emotional wellbeing of midwives in a pandemic: Guidance for RCM.

88. Gavin, B., et al (2020) Caring for the Psychological Well-being of Healthcare Professionals in the Covid-19 Pandemic Crisis. Irish Medical Journal, 113 (4) p51

89. Asefa, A., Semaan, A., Delvaux, T., Huysmans, E., Galle, A., Sacks, E., Bohren, M.A., Morgan, A., Sadler, M., Vedam, S., Benova, L. The impact of Covid-19 on the provision of respectful maternity care: findings from a global survey of health workers. medRxiv. 2021 Jan 1.

90. González-Timoneda, A., Hernández, V.H., Moya, S.P., Blazquez, R.A. Experiences and attitudes of midwives during the birth of a pregnant woman with COVID-19 infection: A qualitative study. Women and Birth. 2021 Sep 1;34(5):465-72.

91. Holton, S., Wynter, K., Trueman, M., Bruce, S., Sweeney, S., Crowe, S., Dabscheck, A., Eleftheriou, P., Booth, S., Hitch, D., Said, C.M. Psychological well-being of Australian hospital clinical staff during the COVID-19 pandemic. Australian Health Review. 2020 Oct 9;45(3):297-305.

92. Yörük, S., Güler, D. The relationship between psychological resilience, burnout, stress, and sociodemographic factors with depression in nurses and midwives during the COVID-19 pandemic: A cross-sectional study in Turkey. Perspectives in Psychiatric Care. 2021 Jan;57(1):390-8.

93. hsib-kqcco125-media.s3.amazonaws.com/assets/documents/HSIB_ Maternal_Death_Report_V13.pdf

94. hsib-kqcco125-media.s3.amazonaws.com/assets/documents/HSIB_ Intrapartum_Stillbirth_Report_web.pdf

CHAPTER 3: GIVING BIRTH WHILE POSITIVE FOR COVID-19

1. www.who.int/emergencies/diseases/novel-coronavirus-2019/question-and-answers-hub/q-a-detail/q-a-on-Covid-19-and-breastfeeding

2. Cleveland, L., Hill, C.M., Pulse, W.S., DiCioccio, H.C., Field, T., White-Traut, R. Systematic review of skin-to-skin care for full-term, healthy newborns. *Journal of Obstetric, Gynecologic & Neonatal Nursing.* 2017 Nov 1;46(6):857-69.

3. Crenshaw, J.T. Healthy birth practice #6: Keep mother and baby together—It's best for mother, baby, and breastfeeding. *The Journal of Perinatal Education.* 2014 Jan 1;23(4):211-7.

4. Victora, C.G., Bahl, R., Barros, A.J., França, G.V., Horton, S., Krasevec, J., Murch, S., Sankar, M.J., Walker, N., Rollins, N.C., Group, T.L. Breastfeeding in the 21st century: epidemiology, mechanisms, and life-long effect. *The Lancet.* 2016 Jan 30;387(10017):475-90.

REFERENCES

5. Chambers, C., Krogstad, P., Bertrand, K., Contreras, D., Tobin, N.H., Bode, L., Aldrovandi, G. Evaluation for SARS-CoV-2 in breast milk from 18 infected women. *JAMA*. 2020 Oct 6;324(13):1347-8.

6. Yang, Y., Brandon, D., Lu, H., Cong, X. (2019). Breastfeeding experiences and perspectives on support among Chinese mothers separated from their hospitalized preterm infants: A qualitative study. *International Breastfeeding Journal*, 14(1),

7. Gribble, K., Marinelli, K.A., Tomori, C., Gross, M.S. Implications of the Covid-19 pandemic response for breastfeeding, maternal caregiving capacity and infant mental health. *Journal of Human Lactation*. 2020 Nov;36(4):591-603.

8. Hoang, D.V., Cashin, J., Gribble, K., Marinelli, K., Mathisen, R. Misalignment of global Covid-19 breastfeeding and newborn care guidelines with World Health Organization recommendations. *BMJ Nutrition, Prevention & Health*. 2020 Dec;3(2):339.

9. AAP. (2020) AAP updates guidance on newborns whose mothers have suspected or confirmed Covid-19 www.aappublications.org/news/2020/05/21/Covid19newborn052120

10. Griffin, I., Benarba, F., Peters, C., Oyelese, Y., Murphy, T., Contreras, D., Gagliardo, C., Nwaobasi-Iwuh, E., DiPentima, M.C., Schenkman, A. The impact of Covid-19 infection on labor and delivery, newborn nursery, and neonatal intensive care unit: prospective observational data from a single hospital system. *American Journal of Perinatology*. 2020 Aug;37(10):1022-30.

11. Tomori, C., Gribble, K., Palmquist, A.E., Ververs, M.T., Gross, M.S. When separation is not the answer: Breastfeeding mothers and infants affected by Covid-19. *Maternal & Child Nutrition*. 2020 Oct;16(4):e13033.

12. Popofsky, S., Noor, A., Leavens-Maurer, J., Quintos-Alagheband, M.L., Mock, A., Vinci, A., Magri, E., Akerman, M., Noyola, E., Rigaud, M., Pak, B. Impact of maternal severe acute respiratory syndrome coronavirus 2 detection on breastfeeding due to infant separation at birth. *The Journal of Pediatrics*. 2020 Nov 1;226:64-70.

13. Del Río, R., Pérez, E.D., Gabriel, M.M., Neo, C.R. Multi-centre study showed reduced compliance with the World Health Organization recommendations on exclusive breastfeeding during Covid-19. *Acta Paediatr Int J Paediatr*. 2020 Jan 1.

14. Bartick, M.C., Valdés, V., Giusti, A., Chapin, E.M., Bhana, N.B., Hernández-Aguilar, M.T., ... & Feldman-Winter, L. (2021). Maternal and Infant Outcomes Associated with Maternity Practices Related to Covid-19: The Covid Mothers Study. *Breastfeeding Medicine*.

15. Afif, E.K., Jain, A., Lewandowski, A.J., Levy, P.T. Preventing disease in the 21st century: early breast milk exposure and later cardiovascular health in premature infants. *Pediatric Research*. 2020 Jan;87(2):385-90.

16. Briere, C.E., McGrath, J., Cong, X., Cusson, R. An integrative review of factors that influence breastfeeding duration for premature infants after NICU hospitalization. *Journal of Obstetric, Gynecologic & Neonatal Nursing*. 2014 May 1;43(3):272-81.

17. Rollins, N., Minckas, N., Jehan, F., Lodha, R., Raiten, D., Thorne, C., Van

de Perre, P., Ververs, M., Walker, N., Bahl, R., Victora, C.G. A public health approach for deciding policy on infant feeding and mother–infant contact in the context of Covid-19. *The Lancet Global Health*. 2021 Feb 22.

18. Fumagalli, S., Ornaghi, S., Borrelli, S., Vergani, P., Nespoli, A. The experiences of childbearing women who tested positive to Covid-19 during the pandemic in northern Italy. *Women and Birth*. 2021 Jan 9.

19. Peng, S., Zhang, Y., Liu, H., Huang, X., Noble, D.J., Yang, L., Lu, W., Luo, Y., Zhu, H., Cao, L., Liu, C. A multi-center survey on the postpartum mental health of mothers and attachment to their neonates during Covid-19 in Hubei Province of China. *Annals of Translational Medicine*. 2021 Mar;9(5).

20. Mayopoulos, G.A., Ein-Dor, T., Li, K.G., Chan, S.J., Dekel, S. Covid-19 positivity associated with traumatic stress response to childbirth and no visitors and infant separation in the hospital. *Scientific Reports*. 2021 Jun 29;11(1):1-8.

21. Chinn, J., Sedighim, S., Kirby, K.A., Hohmann, S., Hameed, A.B., Jolley, J., Nguyen, N.T. Characteristics and Outcomes of Women With Covid-19 Giving Birth at US Academic Centers During the Covid-19 Pandemic. *JAMA Network Open*. 2021 Aug 2;4(8):e2120456-.

22. González-Timoneda, A., Hernández, V.H., Moya, S.P., Blazquez, R.A. Experiences and attitudes of midwives during the birth of a pregnant woman with Covid-19 infection: A qualitative study. *Women and Birth*. 2020 Dec 9.

23. Nespoli, A., Ornaghi, S., Borrelli, S., Vergani, P., Fumagalli, S. Lived experiences of the partners of Covid-19 positive childbearing women: A qualitative study. *Women and Birth*. 2021 Aug 2.

CHAPTER 4: EXPERIENCING PREGNANCY COMPLICATIONS DURING THE PANDEMIC

1.   Shin, H., White-Traut, R. The conceptual structure of transition to motherhood in the neonatal intensive care unit. *Journal of Advanced Nursing*. 2007 Apr 1;58(1):90-94

2.   Flacking, R., Ewald, U., Starrin, B. 'I wanted to do a good job': experiences of 'becoming a mother' and breastfeeding in mothers of very preterm infants after discharge from a neonatal unit. *Social Science & Medicine*. 2007 Jun 30;64(12):2405-16.

3.   Cong, S., Wang, R., Fan, X., Song, X., Sha, L., Zhu, Z., Zhou, H., Liu, Y., Zhang, A. Skin-to-skin contact to improve premature mothers' anxiety and stress state: A meta-analysis. *Maternal & Child Nutrition*. 2021 Jul 13:e13245.

4.   Campbell-Yeo, M.L., Disher, T.C., Benoit, B.L., et al. Understanding kangaroo care and its benefits to preterm infants. *Pediatr Health Med Ther*. 2015;6:15–32.

5.   Caskey, M., Stephens, B., Tucker, R., Vohr, B. Importance of parent talk on the development of preterm infant vocalizations. *Pediatrics*. 2011;128:910–16.

6.   Reynolds, L.C., Duncan, M.M., Smith, G.C., Mathur, A., Neil, J., Inder, T., Pineda, R.G. Parental presence and holding in the neonatal intensive care unit and associations with early neurobehavior. *Journal of*

Perinatology. 2013 Aug;33(8):636-41.

7. Liu, J., Bann, C., Lester, B., Tronick, E., Das, A., Lagasse, L. *et al.* Neonatal neurobehavior predicts medical and behavioral outcome. *Pediatrics* 2010; **125** (1): e90–e98.

8. Dewey, K.G. (2001). Maternal and fetal stress are associated with impaired lactogenesis in humans. *The Journal of Nutrition, 131*(11), 3012S-3015S.

9. Cuttini, M., Croci, I., Toome, L., Rodrigues, C., Wilson, E., Bonet, M., Gadzinowski, J., Di Lallo, D., Herich, L.C., Zeitlin, J. Breastfeeding outcomes in European NICUs: impact of parental visiting policies. *Archives of Disease in Childhood-Fetal and Neonatal Edition.* 2019 Mar 1;104(2):F151-8.

10. *Covid-19 – guidance for neonatal settings* Royal College of Paediatrics & Child Health, 2020. Available: www.rcpch.ac.uk/resources/ Covid-19-guidance-neonatal-settings#parents-and-visitors-to-nnu

11. *Frequently Asked Questions within Neonatal Services: A BAPM supplement to RCPCH guidance*, 2020. Available: hubble-live-assets.s3.amazonaws.com/bapm/redactor2_assets/files/561/Covid-FAQs_5.7.20.docx. pdf

12. Bliss *Bliss statement: Covid-19 and parental involvement on neonatal units*, 2020

13. Kostenzer, J., Hoffmann, J., von Rosenstiel-Pulver, C., Walsh, A., Zimmermann, L.J., Mader, S. Neonatal care during the Covid-19 pandemic – a global survey of parents' experiences regarding infant and family-centred developmental care. *EClinicalMedicine.* 2021 Sep 1;39:101056.

14. Sanders, J., Blaylock, R. 'Anxious and traumatised': users' experiences of maternity care in the UK during the Covid-19 pandemic. *Midwifery.* 2021 Jun 18:103069.

15. Bembich, S., Tripani, A., Mastromarino, S., Di Risio, G., Castelpietra, E., Risso, F.M. Parents experiencing NICU visit restrictions due to Covid-19 pandemic. *Acta Paediatrica* (Oslo, Norway: 1992). 2020 Oct 16.

16. Vance, A.J., Malin, K.J., Shuman, C.J., Moore, T.A. Parent Experience of Neonatal Hospitalization during the Covid-19 Pandemic. B009 Patient, Family, and Provider Experiences in Critical Care and Chronic Patient Management 2021 May (pp. A1083-A1083). American Thoracic Society.

17. Bin-Nun, A., Palmor-Haspal, S., Mimouni, F.B., Kasirer, Y., Hammerman, C., Tuval-Moshiach, R. Infant delivery and maternal stress during the Covid-19 pandemic: a comparison of the well-baby versus neonatal intensive care environments. *Journal of Perinatology.* 2021 May 13:1-7.

18. Muniraman, H., Ali, M., Cawley, P., Hillyer, J., Heathcote, A., Ponnusamy, V., Coleman, Z., Hammonds, K., Raiyani, C., Gait-Carr, E., Myers, S. Parental perceptions of the impact of neonatal unit visitation policies during Covid-19 pandemic. *BMJ Paediatrics Open.* 2020;4(1).

19. Brown, A., Shenker, N. Experiences of breastfeeding during Covid-19: Lessons for future practical and emotional support. *Maternal & Child Nutrition.* 2021 Jan;17(1):e13088.

20. Gunes, A.O., Dincer, E., Karadag, N., Topcuoglu, S., Karatekin, G. Effects

of Covid-19 pandemic on breastfeeding rates in a neonatal intensive care unit. *Journal of Perinatal Medicine.* 2021 May 1;49(4):500-5

21. Garfield, C.F., Lee, Y.S., Warner-Shifflett, L., Christie, R., Jackson, K.L., Miller, E. Maternal and paternal depression symptoms during NICU stay and transition home. *Pediatrics.* 2021 Aug 1;148(2).

22. Smorti, M., Ponti, L., Simoncini, T., Mannella, P., Bottone, P., Pancetti, F., Marzetti, F., Mauri, G., Gemignani, A. Pregnancy after miscarriage in primiparae and multiparae: implications for women's psychological well-being. *Journal of Reproductive and Infant Psychology.* 2021 Aug 8;39(4):371-81.

23. Krosch, D.J., & Shakespeare-Finch, J. (2017). Grief, traumatic stress, and posttraumatic growth in women who have experienced pregnancy loss. *Psychological Trauma: Theory, Research, Practice and Policy,* 9(4), 425–433

24. deMontigny, F., Verdon, C., Meunier, S., & Dubeau, D. (2017). Women's persistent depressive and perinatal grief symptoms following a miscarriage: The role of childlessness and satisfaction with healthcare services. *Archives of Womens Mental Health,* 20, 655-662.

25. Dong, X., Guopeng, L., Lui, C., Kong, L., Fang, Y., Kang, X., & Li, P. (2017). The mediating role of resilience in the relationship between social support and posttraumatic growth among colorectal cancer survivors with permanent intestinal ostomies: A structural equation model analysis. *European Journal of Oncology Nursing, 29,* 47-52

26. Miller, M., Iyer, D.D., Hawkins, C., Freedle, A. The Impact of Covid-19 Pandemic on Women's Adjustment Following Pregnancy Loss: Brief Report.

27. www.lindenwood.edu/files/resources/pregnancy-loss-Covid-19.pdf

28. Deka, P.K., Sarma, S. Psychological aspects of infertility. *Br J Med Pract* 2010;3:a336

29. Boivin, J., Harrison, C., Mathur, R., Burns, G., Pericleous-Smith, A., Gameiro, S. Patient experiences of fertility clinic closure during the Covid-19 pandemic: appraisals, coping and emotions. *Human Reproduction.* 2020 Nov;35(11):2556-66.

30. Turcoy, J.M., Hercz, D., D'Alton, M., Forman, E.J, Williams, Z.R.A., 2020. The emotional impact of the ASRM guidelines on fertility patients during the Covid-19 pandemic. https://doi.org/ 10.1101/2020.03.29.20046631

31. Barra, F., La Rosa, V.L., Vitale, S.G., Commodari, E., Altieri, M., Scala, C., Ferrero, S. Psychological status of infertile patients who had in vitro fertilization treatment interrupted or postponed due to Covid-19 pandemic: a cross-sectional study. *Journal of Psychosomatic Obstetrics & Gynecology.* 2021 Jan 9:1-8.

32. Ben-Kimhy, R., Youngster, M., Medina-Artom, T.R., Avraham, S., Gat, I., Marom Haham, L., Hourvitz, A., Kedem, A. Fertility patients under Covid-19: attitudes, perceptions and psychological reactions. *Human Reproduction.* 2020 Dec;35(12):2774-83.

33. Haham, L.M., Youngster, M., Shani, A.K., Yee, S., Ben-Kimhy, R., Medina-Artom, T.R., Hourvitz, A., Kedem, A., Librach, C. Suspension of fertility treatment during the Covid-19 pandemic: views, emotional reactions

and psychological distress among women undergoing fertility treatment. *Reproductive Biomedicine Online.* 2021 Apr 1;42(4):849-58.

CHAPTER 5: POSTNATAL CARE DURING THE PANDEMIC

1. Winson, N. (2017). Transition to motherhood. In *The social context of birth* (pp. 141-155). Routledge.
2. Harries, V., & Brown, A. (2017). The association between use of infant parenting books that promote strict routines, and maternal depression, self-efficacy, and parenting confidence. *Early Child Development and Care.*
3. Lee, K., Vasileiou, K., & Barnett, J. (2019). 'Lonely within the mother': An exploratory study of first-time mothers' experiences of loneliness. *Journal of Health Psychology, 24*(10), 1334-1344.
4. Feng, Z., & Savani, K. (2020). Covid-19 created a gender gap in perceived work productivity and job satisfaction: implications for dual-career parents working from home. *Gender in Management: An International Journal.* Vol. 35 No. 7/8, 2020 pp. 719-736
5. Henderson, J., Carson, C., Redshaw, M. Impact of preterm birth on maternal well-being and women's perceptions of their baby: a population-based survey. *BMJ Open.* 2016 Oct 1;6(10):e012676.
6. www.gov.uk/government/publications/healthy-child-programme-pregnancy-and-the-first-5-years-of-life
7. Alderdice, F., McNeill, J., Lynn, F. A systematic review of systematic reviews of interventions to improve maternal mental health and well-being. *Midwifery.* 2013 Apr 1;29(4):389-99.
8. Gilmer, C., Buchan, J.L., Letourneau, N., Bennett, C.T., Shanker, S.G., Fenwick, A., & Smith-Chant, B. (2016). Parent education interventions designed to support the transition to parenthood: A realist review. *International Journal of Nursing Studies, 59*, 118-133.
9. Davies, S.C., Bick, D., MacArthur, C., Knight, M., et al. (2015) Post-pregnancy care: missed opportunities in the reproductive years. In *Annual report of the Chief Medical Officer*, 2014. The health of the 51%: women, ed Davies, S.C. (Department of Health, London)
10. www.nursingtimes.net/news/children/survey-reveals-pressures-faced-by-health-visitors-since-Covid-19-23-12-2020/
11. allcatsrgrey.org.uk/wp/download/public_health/health_visiting/State-of-Health-Visiting-survey-2020-FINAL-VERSION-18.12.20.pdf
12. discovery.ucl.ac.uk/id/eprint/10106430/8/Conti_Dow_The%20impacts%20of%20Covid-19%20on%20Health%20Visiting%20in%20England%20250920.pdf
13. www.communitycare.co.uk/2020/11/10/Covid-pressure-cooker-behind-20-rise-reports-serious-harm-babies-says-ofsted-head/
14. Sidpra, J., Abomeli, D., Hameed, B., Baker, J., Mankad, K. Rise in the incidence of abusive head trauma during the Covid-19 pandemic. *Archives of Disease in Childhood.* 2021 Mar 1;106(3):e14-.
15. Schmidt, S., Natanson, H. With kids stuck at home, ER doctors see more severe cases of child abuse. *Washington Post.* April 30, 2020. Accessed: May 4, 2020. www.washingtonpost.com/education/2020/04/30/

child-abuse-reports-coronavirus

16. discovery.ucl.ac.uk/id/eprint/10106430/8/Conti_Dow_The%20 impacts%20of%20Covid-19%20on%20Health%20Visiting%20in%20 England%20250920.pdf

17. www.theguardian.com/society/2019/dec/01/ health-visitor-numbers-in-england-fall-by-a-third-under-tories

18. www.england.nhs.uk/coronavirus/wp-content/uploads/ sites/52/2020/03/20200527-Covid-19-restoration-of-community-health-services-change-log.pdf

19. Panda, S., O'Malley, D., Barry, P., Vallejo, N., Smith, V. Women's views and experiences of maternity care during Covid-19 in Ireland: A qualitative descriptive study. *Midwifery*. 2021 Dec 1;103:103092.

20. McKinstry, B., Hammersley, V., Burton, C., Pinnock, H., Elton, R., Dowell, J., Sawdon, N., Heaney, D., Elwyn, G., Sheikh, A. The quality, safety and content of telephone and face-to-face consultations: a comparative study. *BMJ Quality & Safety*. 2010 Aug 1;19(4):298-303.

21. Das, R. Women's experiences of maternity and perinatal mental health services during the first Covid-19 lockdown. *Journal of Health Visiting*. 2021 Jul 2;9(7):297-303.

22. Altman, M.R., Gavin, A.R., Eagen-Torkko, M.K., Kantrowitz-Gordon, I., Khosa, R.M., Mohammed, S.A. Where the system failed: the Covid-19 pandemic's impact on pregnancy and birth care. *Global Qualitative Nursing Research*. 2021

23. Rhodes, A., Kheireddine, S., Smith, A.D. Experiences, Attitudes, and Needs of Users of a Pregnancy and Parenting App (Baby Buddy) During the Covid-19 Pandemic: Mixed Methods Study *JMIR Mhealth Uhealth* 2020;8(12):e23157

24. Marshall, J., Kihlström, L., Buro, A., Chandran, V., Prieto, C., Stein-Elger, R., Koeut-Futch, K., Parish, A., Hood, K. Statewide implementation of virtual perinatal home visiting during Covid-19. *Maternal and Child Health Journal*. 2020 Oct;24(10):1224-30.

25. healthforunder5s.co.uk/sections/foryou/ health-visitors-during-the-coronavirus-outbreak/

26. Driscoll, J., Lorek, A., Kinnear, E., Hutchinson, A. Multi-agency safe-guarding arrangements: overcoming the challenges of Covid-19 measures. *Journal of Children's Services*. 2020 Nov 2.

27. Shelter (2019a) A child becomes homeless in Britain every eight minutes. england.shelter.org.uk/media/press_releases/ articles/a_child_becomes_homeless_in_britain_every_eight_minutes

28. Children's Commissioner for England (2019) Bleak Houses: Tackling the crisis of family homelessness in England. www.childrenscommis-sioner.gov.uk/publication/bleak-houses

29. Dorney-Smith, S., Williams, J., Gladstone, C. Health visiting with home-less families during the Covid-19 pandemic. *Journal of Health Visiting*. 2020 May 2;8(5):190-3.

30. www.local.gov.uk/joint-letter-winter-planning-support-chil-dren-and-families-7-october-2020

31. www.nursingtimes.net/news/public-health/

warning-against-further-health-visitor-and-school-nurse-redeployment-09-10-2020

CHAPTER 6: EXPERIENCES OF INFANT FEEDING DURING THE PANDEMIC

1. www.standard.co.uk/news/uk/desperate-mums-forced-to-pay-ps155-for-ps8-baby-milk-on-ebay-a4391981.html
2. Brown, A., & Shenker, N. (2021). Experiences of breastfeeding during Covid-19: Lessons for future practical and emotional support. *Maternal & Child Nutrition*, 17(1), e13088.
3. *Babies in Lockdown: listening to parents to build back better* (2020). Best Beginnings, Home-Start UK, and the Parent-Infant Foundation UK.
4. Spatz, D.L., Froh, E.B. Birth and breastfeeding in the hospital setting during the Covid-19 pandemic. *MCN: The American Journal of Maternal/Child Nursing*. 2021 Jan 1;46(1):30-5.
5. Panda, S., O'Malley, D., Barry, P., Vallejo, N., Smith, V. Women's views and experiences of maternity care during Covid-19 in Ireland: A qualitative descriptive study. *Midwifery*. 2021 Dec 1;103:103092
6. Zanardo, V., Tortora, D., Guerrini, P., Garani, G., Severino, L., Soldera, G., Straface, G. Infant feeding initiation practices in the context of Covid-19 lockdown. *Early Human Development*. 2021 Jan 1;152:105286.
7. Bartick, M. (2020) Covid-19: Separating infected mothers from newborns: Weighing the risks and benefits. trends. hms.harvard.edu/2020/03/31/Covid-19- separating-infected-mothers-from-newborns-weighing-the-risks-and-benefits/
8. AAP. (2020) AAP updates guidance on newborns whose mothers have suspected or confirmed Covid-19 www.aappublications.org/news/2020/05/21/Covid-19newborn052120
9. World Health Organization Euro. (2020) Covid-19 and breastfeeding: position paper. Available at: www.euro.who.int/__data/assets/pdf_file/0010/437788/breastfeeding-Covid-19.pdf?ua=1
10. Tomori, C., Gribble, K., Palmquist, A.E., Ververs, M.T., & Gross, M.S. (2020). When separation is not the answer: Breastfeeding mothers and infants affected by Covid-19. *Maternal & Child Nutrition*, 16(4), e13033.
11. Groß, R., Conzelmann, C., Müller, J.A., Stenger, S., Steinhart, K., Kirchhoff, F., Münch, J. Detection of SARS-CoV-2 in human breastmilk. *The Lancet*. 2020 Jun 6;395(10239):1757-8.
12. WHO. (2020b) Breastfeeding and Covid-19 www.who.int/publications/i/item/10665332639
13. Lowe, B., Bopp, B. Covid-19 vaginal delivery–a case report. *Australian and New Zealand Journal of Obstetrics and Gynaecology*. 2020 Jun;60(3):465-6.
14. Victora, C.G., Rollins, N.C., Murch, S., Krasevec, J., Bahl, R. Breastfeeding in the 21st century–Authors' reply. *The Lancet*. 2016 May 21;387(10033):2089-90.
15. Brown, A. What do women lose if they are prevented from meeting their breastfeeding goals?. *Clinical Lactation*. 2018 Nov 1;9(4):200-7.
16. Hull, N., Kam, R.L., Gribble, K.D. Providing breastfeeding support during the Covid-19 pandemic: Concerns of mothers who contacted the

Australian Breastfeeding Association. *Breastfeeding Review.* 2020 Nov;28(3):25-35.

17. Snyder, K., Worlton, G. Social support during Covid-19: Perspectives of breastfeeding mothers. *Breastfeeding Medicine.* 2021 Jan 1;16(1):39-45.

18. Moukarzel, S., Del Fresno, M., Bode, L., Daly, A.J. Distance, diffusion and the role of social media in a time of Covid contagion. *Maternal & Child Nutrition.* 2020 Oct;16(4).

19. Karavadra, B., Stockl, A., Prosser-Snelling, E., Simpson, P., Morris, E. Women's perceptions of Covid-19 and their healthcare experiences: a qualitative thematic analysis of a national survey of pregnant women in the United Kingdom. *BMC Pregnancy and Childbirth.* 2020 Dec;20(1):1-8.

20. Trickey, H., Thomson, G., Grant, A., Sanders, J., Mann, M., Murphy, S., Paranjothy, S. A realist review of one-to-one breastfeeding peer support experiments conducted in developed country settings. *Maternal & Child Nutrition.* 2018 Jan;14(1):e12559.

21. McFadden, A., Gavine, A., Renfrew, M.J., Wade, A., Buchanan, P., Taylor, J.L., Veitch, E., Rennie, A.M., Crowther, S.A., Neiman, S., MacGillivray, S. Support for healthy breastfeeding mothers with healthy term babies. *Cochrane Database of Systematic Reviews.* 2017(2).

22. Vazquez-Vazquez, A., Dib, S., Rougeaux, E., Wells, J.C., & Fewtrell, M.S. (2021). The impact of the Covid-19 lockdown on the experiences and feeding practices of new mothers in the UK: Preliminary data from the Covid-19 New Mum Study. *Appetite,* 156, 104985.

23. McAndrew, F., Thompson, J., Fellows, L., Large, A., Speed, M., Renfrew, M.J. *Infant feeding survey 2010.* Leeds: Health and Social Care Information Centre. 2012 Nov 20;2(1).

24. Rollins, N.C., Bhandari, N., Hajeebhoy, N., Horton, S., Lutter, C.K., Martines, J.C., Piwoz, E.G., Richter, L.M., Victora, C.G., Group, T.L. Why invest, and what it will take to improve breastfeeding practices?. *The Lancet.* 2016 Jan 30;387(10017):491-504.

25. Minchin, M., Hons BA. 14 Infant Feeding in History: an Outline. *Breastfeeding and Breast Milk - From Biochemistry to Impact: A Multidisciplinary Introduction.* 2018 Sep 19:219.

26. Brown, A. *Breastfeeding Uncovered: Who really decides how we feed our babies?* 2021. Pinter & Martin.

27. Silverio, S.A., De Backer, K., Easter, A., von Dadelszen, P., Magee, L.A., Sandall, J. Women's experiences of maternity service reconfiguration during the Covid-19 pandemic: A qualitative investigation. *Midwifery.* 2021 Aug 5:103116.

28. Rhodes, A., Kheireddine, S., Smith, A.D. Experiences, Attitudes, and Needs of Users of a Pregnancy and Parenting App (Baby Buddy) During the Covid-19 Pandemic: Mixed Methods Study *JMIR Mhealth Uhealth* 2020;8(12):e23157

29. Ceulemans, M.; Hompes, T.; Foulon, V. Mental health status of pregnant and breastfeeding women during the Covid-19 pandemic: A call for action. *Int. J. Gynecol. Obs.* **2020**, *151*, 146–147.

30. Ingram, J., Cann, K., Peacock, J., & Potter, B. (2008). Exploring the

barriers to exclusive breastfeeding in black and minority ethnic groups and young mothers in the UK. *Maternal & Child Nutrition, 4*(3), 171-180.

31. www.dailymail.co.uk/news/article-8927847/Formula-milk-firms-bombard- ed-parents-social-media-coronavirus-lockdown.html

32. McCreedy, A., Bird, S., Brown, L.J., Shaw-Stewart, J., & Chen, Y.F. (2018). Effects of maternal caffeine consumption on the breastfed child: a systematic review. *Swiss Medical Weekly,* 148(3940).

33. Haastrup, M.B., Pottegard, A., & Damkier, P. (2014). Alcohol and breastfeeding. *Basic & Clinical Pharmacology & Toxicology,* 114(2), 168-173.

34. Marangoni, F., Cetin, I., Verduci, E., Canzone, G., Giovannini, M., Scollo, P., Corsello, G., Poli, A. Maternal diet and nutrient requirements in pregnancy and breastfeeding. An Italian consensus document. *Nutrients.* 2016 Oct;8(10):629.

35. van Tulleken, C., Wright, C., Brown, A., McCoy, D., & Costello, A. (2020). Marketing of breastmilk substitutes during the Covid-19 pandemic. *The Lancet,* 396(10259), e58.

36. Shenker, N., Aprigio, J., Arslanoglu, S., San San Aye, N., Bærug, A., Yam, N.B., Barnett, D., Bellad, R., Bertino, E., Bethou, A., Bharadva, K. Maintaining safety and service provision in human milk banking: a call to action in response to the Covid-19 pandemic. *The Lancet Child & Adolescent Health.* 2020 Jul 1;4(7):484-5.

37. heartsmilkbank.org/faqs

38. www.who.int/elena/titles/hiv_infant_feeding/en/

39. Marinelli, K.A. International perspectives concerning donor milk banking during the SARS-CoV-2 (Covid-19) pandemic. *Journal of Human Lactation.* 2020 Aug;36(3):492-7.

40. Sachdeva, R.C., Jain, S., Mukherjee, S., Singh, J. Ensuring exclusive human milk diet for all babies in Covid-19 times. *Indian Pediatrics.* 2020 Aug;57(8):730-3.

41. Chambers, C., Krogstad, P., Bertrand, K., Conteras, D., Bode, L., Tobin, N., et al. Preprint: Evaluation of SARS-CoV-2 in breastmilk from 18 infected women. 2020.

42. World Health Organization. (2020a). Breastfeeding advice during the Covid-19 outbreak. www.emro.who.int/nutrition/nutrition-infocus/ breastfeeding-advice-during-Covid-19-outbreak.html

43. Shenker, N., Staff, M., Vickers, A., Aprigio, J., Tiwari, S., Nangia, S., Sachdeva, R.C., Clifford, V., Coutsoudis, A., Reimers, P., Israel-Ballard, K. Maintaining human milk bank services throughout the Covid-19 pandemic: A global response. *Maternal & Child Nutrition.* 2021 Jan 6:e13131.

CHAPTER 7: PANDEMIC POSTNATAL MENTAL HEALTH

1. Winson, N. (2017). Transition to motherhood. In *The social context of birth* (pp. 141-155). Routledge

2. Don, B.P., Chong, A., Biehle, S.N., Gordon, A., & Mickelson, K.D. (2014). Anxiety across the transition to parenthood: change trajectories among low-risk parents. *Anxiety, Stress, & Coping, 27*(6), 633-649

3. Nelson, S.K., Kushlev, K., & Lyubomirsky, S. (2014). The pains and pleasures of parenting: When, why, and how is parenthood associated with

more or less well-being?. *Psychological bulletin, 140*(3), 846.

4. Milgrom, J., Gemmill, A.W., Bilszta, J.L., Hayes, B., Barnett, B., Brooks, J., ... & Buist, A. (2008). Antenatal risk factors for postnatal depression: a large prospective study. *Journal of Affective Disorders, 108*(1-2), 147-157.

5. Philpott, L.F., Leahy-Warren, P., FitzGerald, S., Savage, E. (2017) . Stress in fathers in the perinatal period: A systematic review. *Midwifery*. 2, 55: 113-127.

6. Paulson, J., Bazemore, S. (2010). Prenatal and postpartum depression in fathers and its association with maternal depression: a meta-analysis. *JAMA*. 2010; 303(19): 1961-1969.

7. Stadtlander L. (2015) Paternal postpartum depression. *International Journal of Childbirth Education*. 30(2): 11–13.

8. Parfitt, Y., & Ayers, S. (2012). Postnatal mental health and parenting: The importance of parental anger. *Infant Mental Health Journal, 33*(4), 400-410.

9. Ou, C.H., & Hall, W.A. (2018). Anger in the context of postnatal depression: An integrative review. *Birth, 45*(4), 336-346.

10. Tsivos, Z.L., Calam, R., Sanders, M.R., & Wittkowski, A. (2015). Interventions for postnatal depression assessing the mother–infant relationship and child developmental outcomes: a systematic review. *International Journal of Women's Health, 7*, 429.

11. Myers, S., & Johns, S.E. (2018). Postnatal depression is associated with detrimental life-long and multi-generational impacts on relationship quality. *PeerJ, 6*, e4305.

12. McCabe, J.E., Wickberg, B., Deberg, J., Davila, R.C., & Segre, L. S. (2021). Listening Visits for maternal depression: a meta-analysis. *Archives of Women's Mental Health*, 1-9.

13. Shakespeare, J., Blake, F., & Garcia, J. (2006). How do women with post-natal depression experience listening visits in primary care? A qualitative interview study. *Journal of Reproductive and Infant Psychology, 24*(02), 149-162.

14. Riley, V., Ellis, N., Mackay, L., Taylor, J. The impact of Covid-19 restrictions on women's pregnancy and postpartum experience in England: A qualitative exploration. *Midwifery*. 2021 Jun 5.

15. Sweet, L., Bradfield, Z., Vasilevski, V., Wynter, K., Hauck, Y., Kuliukas, L., Homer, C.S., Szabo, R.A., Wilson, A.N. Becoming a mother in the 'new' social world in Australia during the first wave of the Covid-19 pandemic. *Midwifery*. 2021 Jul 1;98:102996.

16. Rhodes, A., Kheireddine, S., Smith, A.D. Experiences, Attitudes, and Needs of Users of a Pregnancy and Parenting App (Baby Buddy) During the Covid-19 Pandemic: Mixed Methods Study *JMIR Mhealth Uhealth* 2020;8(12):e23157

17. Dib, S., Rougeaux, E., Vázquez-Vázquez, A., Wells, J.C., & Fewtrell, M. (2020). The impact of the Covid-19 lockdown on maternal mental health and coping in the UK: Data from the Covid-19 New Mum Study. *medRxiv*.

18. *Babies in Lockdown: listening to parents to build back better* (2020). Best Begin- nings, Home-Start UK, and the Parent-Infant Foundation UK.

19. Davenport, M.H., Meyer, S., Meah, V.L., Strynadka, M.C., & Khurana,

R. (2020). Moms are not ok: Covid-19 and maternal mental health. *Frontiers in Global Women's Health*, 1, 1.

20. Fallon, V., Davies, S.M., Silverio, S.A., Jackson, L., De Pascalis, L., & Harrold, J.A. (2021). Psychosocial experiences of postnatal women during the Covid-19 pandemic. A UK-wide study of prevalence rates and risk factors for clinically relevant depression and anxiety. *Journal of Psychiatric Research*.

21. Chivers, B.R., Garad, R.M., Boyle, J.A., Skouteris, H., Teede, H.J., Harrison, C.L. Perinatal distress during Covid-19: thematic analysis of an online parenting forum. *Journal of Medical Internet Research*. 2020;22(9):e22002.

22. Silverio, S.A., De Backer, K., Easter, A., von Dadelszen, P., Magee, L.A., Sandall, J. Women's experiences of maternity service reconfiguration during the Covid-19 pandemic: A qualitative investigation. *Midwifery*. 2021 Aug 5:103116.

23. Das, R. Women's experiences of maternity and perinatal mental health services during the first Covid-19 lockdown. *Journal of Health Visiting*. 2021 Jul 2;9(7):297-303.

24. Adisa, T.A., Aiyenitaju, O., & Adekoya, O.D. (2021). The work–family balance of British working women during the Covid-19 pandemic. *Journal of Work Applied Management*.

25. Collins, C., Landivar, L.C., Ruppanner, L., & Scarborough, W.J. (2021). Covid-19 and the gender gap in work hours. *Gender, Work & Organization*, 28, 101-112.

26. Khan, Z. (2021). Ethnic health inequalities in the UK's maternity services: a systematic literature review. *British Journal of Midwifery*, 29(2), 100-107.

27. Vahdaninia, M., Simkhada, B., Van Teijlingen, E., Blunt, H., & Mercel-Sanca, A. (2020). Mental health services designed for Black, Asian and Minority Ethnics (BAME) in the UK: a scoping review of case studies. *Mental Health and Social Inclusion*.

28. Brooks, R., Hodkinson, P. Out-of-place: the lack of engagement with parent networks of caregiving fathers of young children. *Families, Relationships and Societies*. 2020 Jul 1;9(2):201-16.

29. Hambidge, S., Cowell, A, Arden-Close, E. Mayers, A., (2021) What kind of man gets depressed after having a baby? *BMC Pregnancy Childbirth*

30. Menzies J. Forgotten fathers: The impact of service reduction during Covid-19. *Journal of Health Visiting*. 2021 Apr 2;9(4):150-3.

31. Hodkinson, P., Das, R. (2021) *New Fathers, Mental Health and Digital Communication*. Palgrave Pivot. Chem, Switzerland.

32. Mayers, A., Hambidge, S., Bryant, O., Arden-Close, E. (2020) Supporting women who develop poor postnatal mental health: what support do fathers receive to support their partner and their own mental health? *BMC Pregnancy Childbirth* 20, 359

33. Recto, P., Lesser, J. Young Hispanic fathers during Covid-19: Balancing parenthood, finding strength, and maintaining hope. *Public Health Nursing*. 2021 May 1.

34. Cameron, E.E., Joyce, K.M., Rollins, K., Roos, L.E. Paternal Depression &

Anxiety During the Covid-19 Pandemic.

35.   Sun, G.Q., Wang, Q., Wang, S.S., Cheng, Y. Risk assessment of paternal depression in relation to partner delivery during Covid-19 pandemic in Wuhan, China. *BMC Psychiatry*. 2021 Dec;21(1):1-8.

36.   Nolvi, S., Karukivi, M., Korja, R., Lindblom, J., Karlsson, L., Karlsson, H. Parental depressive and anxiety symptoms as a response to the Covid-19 pandemic: a birth cohort follow-up study.

37.   Sponton, A. Exploring Covid-19 lockdowns as unexpected paternity leave: One shock, diverse gender ideologies. *Journal of Family Research*. 2021 Aug 12.

CHAPTER 8: THE IMPACT OF LOCKDOWN ON INFANT HEALTH AND DEVELOPMENT

1.   Winnicott, D.W. Primary maternal preoccupation. The maternal lineage: Identification, desire, and transgenerational issues. 1956:59-66.

2.   Rhodes, A., Kheireddine, S., Smith, A.D. Experiences, Attitudes, and Needs of Users of a Pregnancy and Parenting App (Baby Buddy) During the Covid-19 Pandemic: Mixed Methods Study *JMIR Mhealth Uhealth* 2020;8(12):e23157

3.   Silverio, S.A., De Backer, K., Easter, A., von Dadelszen, P., Magee, L.A., Sandall, J. Women's experiences of maternity service reconfiguration during the Covid-19 pandemic: A qualitative investigation. *Midwifery*. 2021 Aug 5:103116.

4.   Public Health England. Emergency department syndromic surveillance system: England, week 16. 2020. assets.publishing.service.gov.uk/government/uploads/system/uploads/attachment_data/file/880759/EDSSSBulletin2020wk16.pdf.

5.   McDonald, H.I., Tessier, E., White, J.M., et al. Early impact of the coronavirus disease (Covid-19) pandemic and physical distancing measures on routine childhood vaccinations in England, January to April 2020. *Euro Surveill* 2020;25:2000848.

6.   www.who.int/news/item/22-05-2020-at-least-80-million-children-under-one-at-risk-of-diseases-such-as-diphtheria-measles-and-polio-as-Covid-19-disrupts-routine-vaccination-efforts-warn-gavi-who-and-unicef

7.   Bell, S., Clarke, R., Paterson, P., Mounier-Jack, S. Parents' and guardians' views and experiences of accessing routine childhood vaccinations during the coronavirus (Covid-19) pandemic: A mixed methods study in England. *PloS one*. 2020 Dec 28;15(12):e0244049.

8.   *Babies in Lockdown: listening to parents to build back better* (2020). Best Begin- nings, Home-Start UK, and the Parent-Infant Foundation UK.

9.   Gonidakis, F., Rabavilas, A.D., Varsou, E., Kreatsas, G., Christodoulou, G.N. A 6-month study of postpartum depression and related factors in Athens Greece. *Comprehensive Psychiatry*. 2008 30;49(3):275-82.

10.   Khushdil, A., Ahmed, Z., Waqar, T., Haque, K.N., Sultana, R., Sughra, U., Ahmed, M., Malik, Q.U. Outcome of Neonates Born to Mothers Who Are Covid-19 Positive; An Observation Cohort Study from Pakistan. 2021 Jan 22.

11.   Patel, R.B., Skaria, S.D., Mansour, M.M., Smaldone, G.C. Respiratory

source control using a surgical mask: an in vitro study. *Journal of Occupational and Environmental Hygiene*. 2016 Jul 2;13(7):569-76.

12. Anfinrud, P., Stadnytskyi, V., Bax, C.E., Bax, A. Visualizing speech-generated oral fluid droplets with laser light scattering. *New England Journal of Medicine*. 2020 May 21;382(21):2061-3.

13. Green, J., Petty, J., Staff, L., Bromley, P., Jones, L. The implications of face masks for babies and families during the Covid-19 pandemic: A discussion paper. *Journal of Neonatal Nursing*. 2020 Oct 29.

14. Harding, C., Aloysius, A., Bell, N., Edney, S., Gordon, Z., Lewis, H., Sweeting, M., Murphy, R. Reflections on Covid-19 and the potential impact on preterm infant feeding and speech, language and communication development. *Journal of Neonatal Nursing*. 2021 Jun 1;27(3):220-2.

15. Zarbatany, L., Lamb, M.E. Social referencing as a function of information source: Mothers versus strangers. *Infant Behavior and Development*. 1985 Jan 1;8(1):25-33

16. Messinger, D.S., Fogel, A., & Dickson, K.L. (2001). All smiles are positive, but some smiles are more positive than others. *Developmental Psychology*, 37(5), 642

17. Gergely, G., & Watson, J.S. (1999). Early socio-emotional development: Contingency perception and the social-biofeedback model. *Early Social Cognition: Understanding Others in the First Months of Life*, 60, 101-136.

18. Simion, F., Giorgio, E.D. Face perception and processing in early infancy: inborn predispositions and developmental changes. *Frontiers in Psychology*. 2015 Jul 9;6:969.

19. Brazelton, T.B., Koslowski, B., Main, M. *The origins of reciprocity: The early mother-infant interaction*.

20. Johnson, M.H., Dziurawiec, S., Ellis, H., Morton, J. Newborns' preferential tracking of face-like stimuli and its subsequent decline. *Cognition*. 1991 Aug 1;40(1-2):1-9.

21. Melinder, A., Forbes, D., Tronick, E., Fikke, L., & Gredebäck, G. (2010). The development of the still-face effect: Mothers do matter. *Infant Behavior and Development*, 33(4), 472-481

22. Puura, K., Leppänen, J., Salmelin, R., Mäntymaa, M., Luoma, I., Latva, R., & Tamminen, T. (2019). Maternal and infant characteristics connected to shared pleasure in dyadic interaction. *Infant Mental Health Journal*, 40(4), 459-478.

23. Flom, R., Bahrick, L.E. The development of infant discrimination of affect in multimodal and unimodal stimulation: The role of intersensory redundancy. *Developmental Psychology*. 2007 Jan;43(1):238.

24. Lalonde, K., Werner, L.A. Infants and adults use visual cues to improve detection and discrimination of speech in noise. *Journal of Speech, Language, and Hearing Research*. 2019 Oct 25;62(10):3860-75.

25. Weikum, W.M., Vouloumanos, A., Navarra, J., Soto-Faraco, S., Sebastián-Gallés, N., Werker, J.F. Visual language discrimination in infancy. *Science*. 2007 May 25;316(5828):1159-.

26. Puura, K., Leppänen, J., Salmelin, R., Mäntymaa, M., Luoma, I., Latva, R., Peltola, M., Lehtimäki, T., Tamminen, T. Maternal and infant characteristics connected to shared pleasure in dyadic interaction. *Infant Mental*

Health Journal. 2019 Jul;40(4):459-78.

27. Singh, L., Tan, A., Quinn, P.C. Infants recognize words spoken through opaque masks but not through clear masks. *Developmental Science.* 2021 May 3.

28. Ruba, A.L., Pollak, S.D. Children's emotion inferences from masked faces: Implications for social interactions during Covid-19. *PloS one.* 2020 Dec 23;15(12):e0243708.

CHAPTER 9: VACCINATION CHAOS FOR PREGNANT AND BREASTFEEDING WOMEN

1. Hare, H., & Womersley, K. (2021). Why were breastfeeding women in the UK denied the Covid-19 vaccine?. *BMJ*, 372.

2. www.bbc.co.uk/news/health-58014779

3. www.standard.co.uk/news/uk/royal-college-of-midwives-government-b945954.html

4. pregnantthenscrewed.com/the-safety-of-pregnant-women/

5. www.irishtimes.com/news/ireland/irish-news/i-hope-we-can-save-even-one-person-widower-urges-vaccination-after-Covid-death-of-wife-after-giving-birth-1.4655880

6. www.england.nhs.uk/2021/07/chief-midwife-urges-pregnant-women-to-get-nhs-Covid-jab/

7. https://www.theguardian.com/world/2021/aug/09/worrying-numbers-of-pregnant-women-in-intensive-care-with-Covid

8. www.theguardian.com/world/2020/dec/20/breastfeeding-mothers-will-not-be- offered-Covid-vaccine-say-regulators

9. Kroger, A.T. (2013). *General recommendations on immunization.* General Recommendations Work Group CDC.

10. Jones, W. *Breastfeeding and medication.* Routledge; 2013 Feb 11.

11. www.who.int/publications/i/item/WHO-2019-nCoV-vaccines-SAGE_recommendation-BNT162b2-2021.1

12. www.assets.publishing.service.gov.uk/government/uploads/system/uploads/attach- ment_data/file/965177/Covid-19_vaccination_programme_guidance_for_healthcare_workers_26_February_2021_v3.4.pdf

13. www.bfmed.org/abm-statement-considerations-for-Covid-19-vaccination-in-lac-tation?fbclid=IwAR1qG7rS66IyTDyDlxGIOrwQsoSqDRuX-WMWnjgBXwhOJu-Sofk13veeT3jl8

14. www.infantrisk.com/Covid-19-vaccine-pregnancy-and-breastfeeding?fbclid=I-wAR030ND0pMXbF76x1zjCzj22HCrGGIUCir CFZ-ijHBFUBOeAECkVJQp-Mds0

15. Friedman, M.R., Kigel, A., Bahar, Y., Yogev, Y., Dror, Y., Many, A., Wine, Y. BNT162b2 Covid-19 mRNA vaccine elicits a rapid and synchronized antibody response in blood and milk of breastfeeding women. *medRxiv.* 2021 Jan 1.

16. Perl, S.H., Uzan-Yulzari, A., Klainer, H., Asiskovich, L., Youngster, M., Rinott, E., Youngster, I. SARS-CoV-2–Specific Antibodies in Breast Milk After Covid-19 Vaccination of Breastfeeding Women. *JAMA.* 2021 May 18;325(19):2013-4.

17. McLaurin-Jiang, S., Garner, C.D., Krutsch, K., Hale, T.W. Maternal and

Child Symptoms Following Covid-19 Vaccination Among Breastfeeding Mothers. *Breastfeeding Medicine*. 2021 Jun 25

18. Baden, L.R., El Sahly, H.M., Essink, B., et al. Efficacy and safety of the mRNA-1273 SARS-CoV-2 vaccine. *N Engl J Med* 2020;384:403–416

19. Bartick, M.C., Valdes, V., Giusti, A., et al. Maternal and infant outcomes associated with maternity practices related to Covid-19: The Covid Mothers Study. *Breastfeed Med* 2021;16:189–199

20. Lawrence, R.A. *Breastfeeding: A Guide for the Medical Profession.* Philadelphia, PA: Elsevier, 2011

21. Vojtek, I., Dieussaert, I., Doherty, T.M. Maternal immunization: where are we now and how to move forward? *Ann Med*. 2018;50:193–208

22. Rasmussen, S.A., Watson, A.K., Kennedy, E.D., Broder, K.R., Jamieson, D.J. Vaccines and pregnancy: past, present, and future. *Semin Fetal Neonatal Med* 2014;19:161–9.

23. Whitehead, C.L., Walker, S.P. Consider pregnancy in Covid-19 therapeutic drug and vaccine trials. *The Lancet*. 2020 May 23;395(10237):e92.

24. Chavan, M., Qureshi, H., Karnati, S., Kollikonda, S. Covid-19 Vaccination in Pregnancy: The Benefits Outweigh the Risks. *Journal of Obstetrics and Gynaecology Canada*. 2021 Jul;43(7):814.

25. Ciapponi, A., Bardach, A., Mazzoni, A., Alconada, T., Anderson, A.S., Argento, F.J., Ballivian, J., Bok, K., Comandé, D., Erbelding, E., Goucher, E. Safety of components and platforms of Covid-19 vaccines considered for use in pregnancy: A rapid review. *Vaccine*. 2021 Aug 13.

26. Vousden, N., Ramakrishnan, R., Bunch, K., Morris, E., Simpson, N., Gale, C., O'Brien, P., Quigley, M., Brocklehurst, P., Kurinczuk, J.J., Knight, M. Impact of SARS-CoV-2 variant on the severity of maternal infection and perinatal outcomes: Data from the UK Obstetric Surveillance System national cohort. *medRxiv*. 2021 Jan 1.

27. Modi, N., Ayres-de-Campos, D., Bancalari, E., Benders, M., Briana, D., Di Renzo, G.C., Fonseca, E.B., Hod, M., Poon, L., Cortes, M.S., Simeoni, U. Equity in coronavirus disease 2019 vaccine development and deployment. *American Journal of Obstetrics and Gynecology*. 2021 May 1;224(5):423-7.

28. Male, V. Are Covid-19 vaccines safe in pregnancy?. *Nature Reviews Immunology*. 2021;21(4):200-1.

29. Pardi, N., Hogan, M.J., Porter, F.W. & Weissman, D. mRNA vaccines — a new era in vaccinology. *Nat. Rev. Drug Discov.* **17**, 261–279 (2018).

30. Cosma, S. et al. Coronavirus disease 2019 and first-trimester spontaneous abortion: a case–control study of 225 pregnant patients. *Am. J. Obstet. Gynecol.*

31. Graham, J.M., Jr Update on the gestational effects of maternal hyperthermia. *Birth Defects Res* 2020;112:943–52

32. Shimabukuro, T.T., Kim, S.Y., Myers, T.R., Moro, P.L., Oduyebo, T., Panagiotakopoulos, L., Marquez, P.L., Olson, C.K., Liu, R., Chang, K.T., Ellington, S.R. Preliminary findings of mRNA Covid-19 vaccine safety in pregnant persons. *New England Journal of Medicine*. 2021 Jun 17;384(24):2273-82.

33. Bookstein Peretz, S., Regev, N., Novick, L., Nachshol, M., Goffer, E.,

Ben-David, A., Asraf, K., Doolman, R., Gal Levin, E., Regev Yochay, G., Yinon, Y. Short-term outcome of pregnant women vaccinated with BNT162b2 mRNA Covid-19 vaccine. *Ultrasound in Obstetrics & Gynecology.* 2021.

34. www.asrm.org/globalassets/asrm/asrm-content/news-and-publications/Covid-19/Covidtaskforceupdate16.pdf

35. Gilbert, P.D., Rudnick, C.A. Newborn antibodies to SARS-CoV-2 detected in cord blood after maternal vaccination. *medRxiv.* 2021 Jan 1.

36. Mithal, L.B., Otero, S., Shanes, E.D., Goldstein, J.A., Miller, E.S. Cord blood antibodies following maternal coronavirus disease 2019 vaccination during pregnancy. *American Journal of Obstetrics & Gynecology.* 2021 Apr 1.

37. Beharier, O., Mayo, R.P., Raz, T., Sacks, K.N., Schreiber, L., Suissa-Cohen, Y., Chen, R., Gomez-Tolub, R., Hadar, E., Gabbay-Benziv, R., Moshkovich, Y.J. Efficient maternal to neonatal transfer of antibodies against SARS-CoV-2 and BNT162b2 mRNA Covid-19 vaccine. *The Journal of Clinical Investigation.* 2021 May 20.

38. Levy, A.T., Singh, S., Riley, L.E., Prabhu, M. Acceptance of Covid-19 vaccination in pregnancy: A survey study. *American Journal of Obstetrics & Gynecology* MFM. 2021 May 18.

39. Skirrow, H., Barnett, S., Bell, S.L., Riaposova, L., Mounier-Jack, S., Kampmann, B., Holder, B. Women's views on accepting Covid-19 vaccination during and after pregnancy, and for their babies: A multi-methods study in the UK. *medRxiv.* 2021 Jan 1.

40. Skjefte, M., Ngirbabul, M., Akeju, O., Escudero, D., Hernandez-Diaz, S., Wyszynski, D.F., Wu, J.W. Covid-19 vaccine acceptance among pregnant women and mothers of young children: results of a survey in 16 countries. *European Journal of Epidemiology.* 2021 Feb;36(2):197-211.

41. Jarrett, C., Wilson, R., O'Leary, M., Eckersberger, E., Larson, H.J. Strategies for addressing vaccine hesitancy–A systematic review. *Vaccine.* 2015 Aug 14;33(34):4180-90.

42. Evans, M.K., Rosenbaum, L., Malina, D., Morrissey, S., Rubin, R.J. Diagnosing and treating systemic racism. *N Engl J Med.* 2020;383:274-276.

43. Jaiswal, J. Whose responsibility is it to dismantle medical mistrust? Future directions for researchers and health care providers. *Behav Med.* 2019;45(2):188-196

44. Jamison, A.M., Quinn, S.C., Freimuth, V.S. 'You don't trust a government vaccine': Narratives of institutional trust and influenza vaccination among African American and white adults. *Soc Sci Med.* 2019;221:87-94.

CHAPTER 10: MOVING FORWARD

1. *Babies in Lockdown: listening to parents to build back better* (2020). Best Beginnings, Home-Start UK, and the Parent-Infant Foundation UK.

2. committees.parliament.uk/publications/7477/documents/78447/default

3. Chiumento, A., Baines, P., Redhead, C., Fovargue, S., Draper, H., Frith, L. Which ethical values underpin England's National Health Service reset

of paediatric and maternity services following Covid-19: a rapid review. *BMJ Open.* 2021 Jun 1;11(6):e049214.

4. publications.parliament.uk/pa/cm5801/cmselect/cmpetitions/526/52606.htm#_idTextAnchor016

5. allcatsrgrey.org.uk/wp/download/public_health/health_visiting/State-of-Health-Visiting-survey-2020-FINAL-VERSION-18.12.20.pdf

6. ihv.org.uk/our-work/publications-reports/health-visiting-during-Covid-19-an-ihv-report/

7. https://discovery.dundee.ac.uk/ws/files/50187305/rcm_supporting_the_emotional_wellbeing_of_midwives_during_a_pandemic_v1_submitted_to_rcm_mrd.pdf

8. ihv.org.uk/wp-content/uploads/2021/07/Health-visiting-making-history-case-studies-FINAL-VERSION-updated-14.7.21.pdf

9. www.rcm.org.uk/media-releases/2021/september/rcm-warns-of-midwife-exodus-as-maternity-staffing-crisis-grows/

10. nationalmaternityvoices.org.uk/wp-content/uploads/2020/05/Select-comm-evidence-april-20-final.pdf

IF YOU'RE READING THIS AS A NEW PARENT

1. theconversation.com/how-to-bond-with-your-baby-if-you-were-separated-during-the-pandemic-160830

INDEX